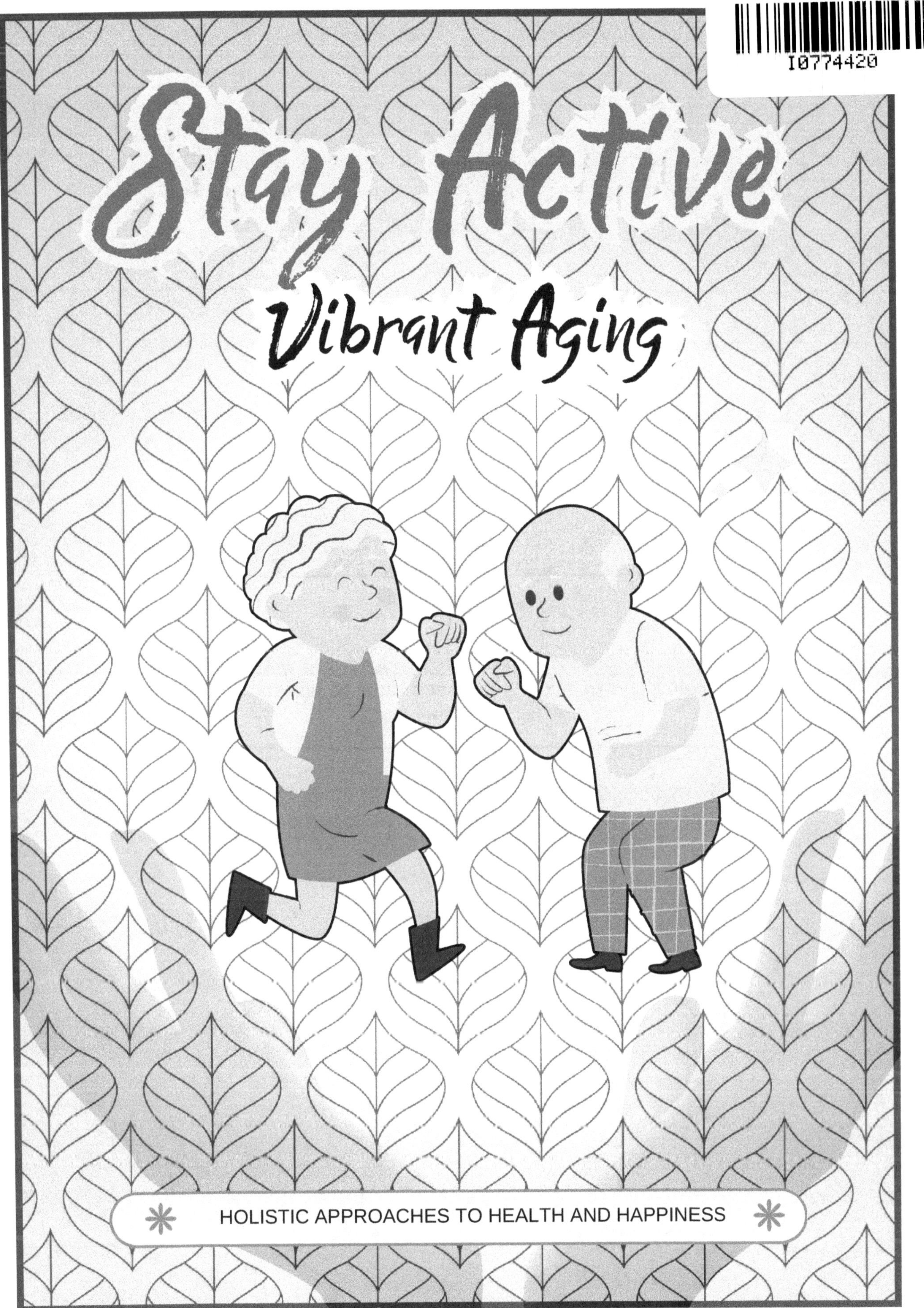

Stay Active
Vibrant Aging
HOLISTIC APPROACHES TO HEALTH AND HAPPINESS

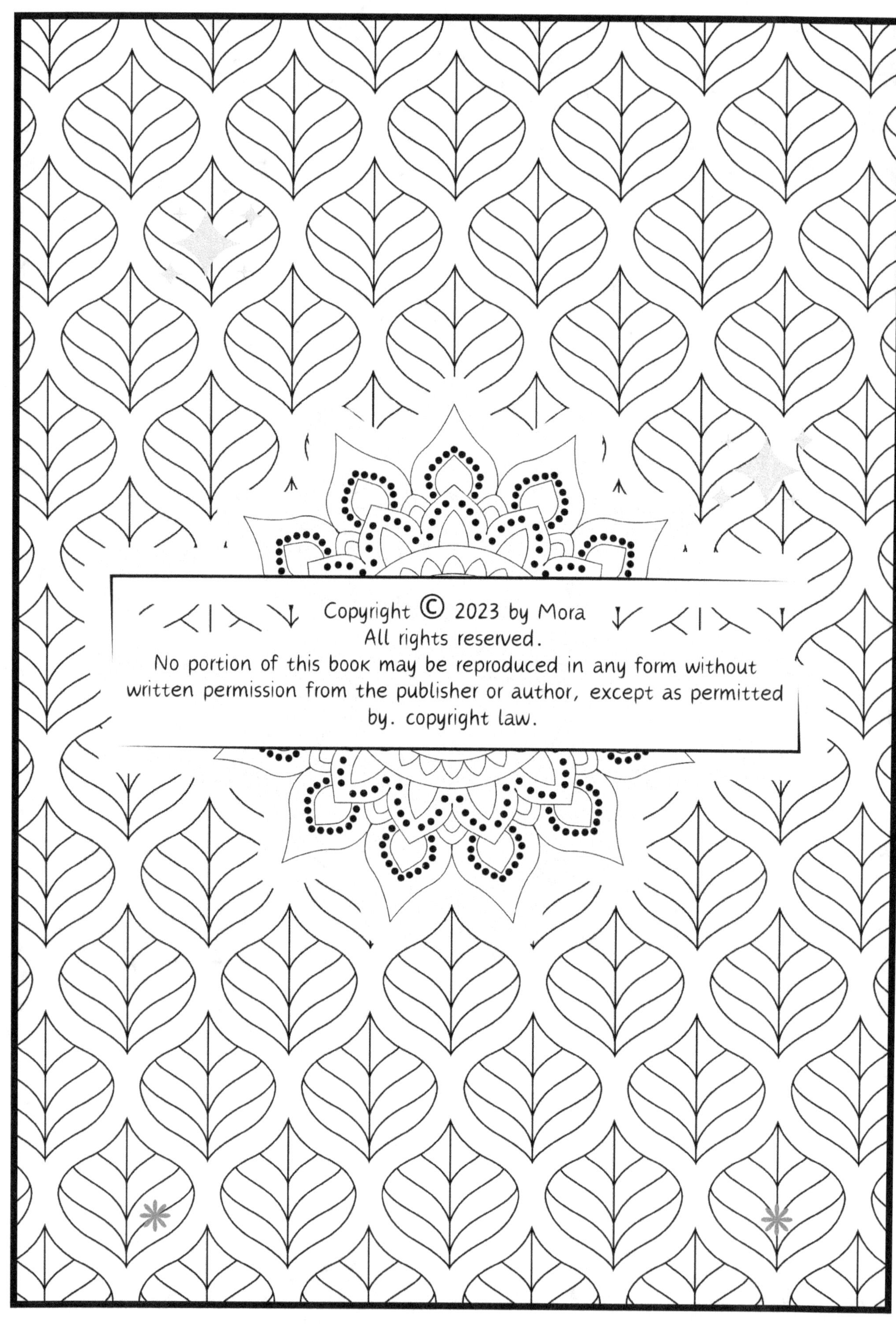

Introduction to Physical Chalenges in Aging

As we age, our bodies undergo natural changes that can have an impact on our physical function and overall health. Physical challenges such as chronic
pain, mobility issues, vision and hearing impairments, and loss of independence can impact daily function and quality of life. In this chapter, we will explore the physical challenges that older adults may face and their impact on daily life.

Chronic Pain

Chronic pain is a common physical challenge that can impact daily function and quality of life. Chronic pain can be caused by a variety of conditions, including arthritis, neuropathy, and back pain. Chronic pain can limit physical activity, sleep quality, and overall well-being.

Mobility Issues

Mobility issues such as difficulty walking, balance problems,

and falls can impact daily function and increase the risk of injury. Mobility issues can be caused by a variety of conditions, including osteoporosis, arthritis, and stroke.

Vision and Hearing Impairments

Vision and hearing impairments can impact daily communication, mobility, and overall well-being. Vision and hearing impairments can be caused by a variety of conditions, including age-related macular degeneration, cataracts, and hearing loss.

Loss of Independence

Loss of independence can impact daily function and overall quality of life. Loss of independence can be caused by a variety of factors, including physical challenges, cognitive decline, and social isolation.

Impact on Daily Life

Physical challenges can impact daily life in many ways. They can limit physical activity, reduce social engagement, and increase the risk of falls and other injuries. Physical challenges can also impact mental health, causing depression, anxiety, and social isolation.

Coping with Physical Challenges

Coping with physical challenges is an essential part of the aging process. Strategies for coping with physical challenges include lifestyle changes such as exercise and a healthy diet, assistive technology such as mobility aids and adaptive equipment, social support from friends and family members, medications and therapies, and coping strategies for managing loss and grief.

Conclusion

Physical challenges are a natural part of the aging process, but they do not have to limit one's ability to enjoy life. By understanding the physical challenges that may arise as we age and the impact they can have on daily life, we can take

proactive steps to manage these challenges and maintain our independence, physical function, and overall well-being. With the right mindset, support, and resources, aging can be a fulfilling and enjoyable journey

Stay Active:

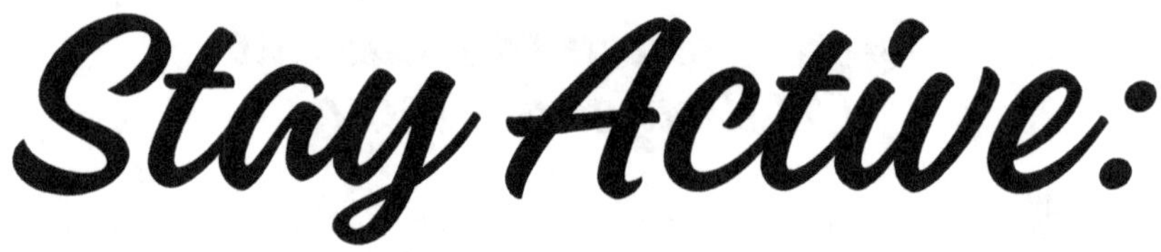

- Engage in regular physical activity, including both aerobic exercises (walking, swimming) and strength training to maintain muscle mass and flexibility.
- Consult with a healthcare professional before starting any new exercise regimen, especially if you have existing health conditions.

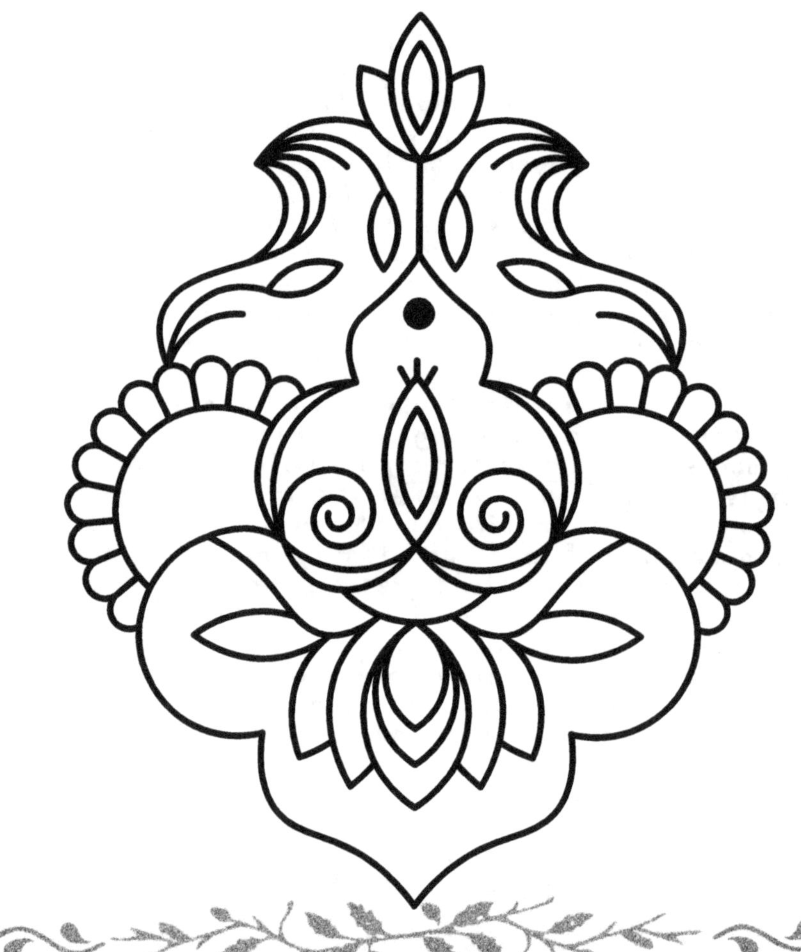

Healthy Diet:

- Adopt a balanced and nutritious diet rich in fruits, vegetables, whole grains, and lean proteins.
- Stay hydrated to support overall health, including joint and muscle function.

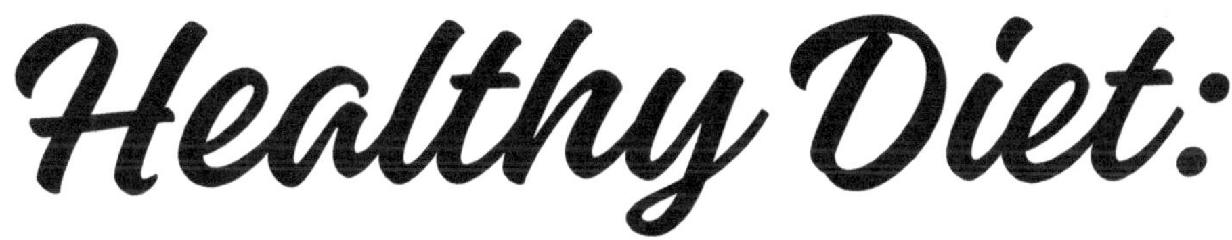

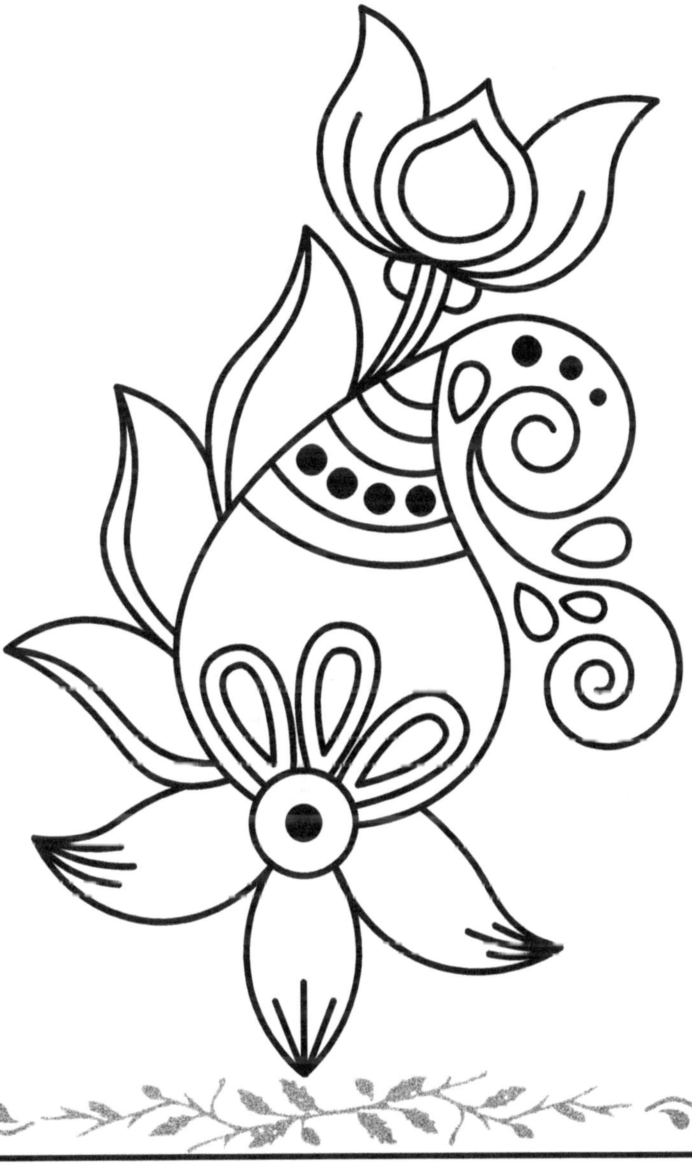

Regular Health Check-ups:

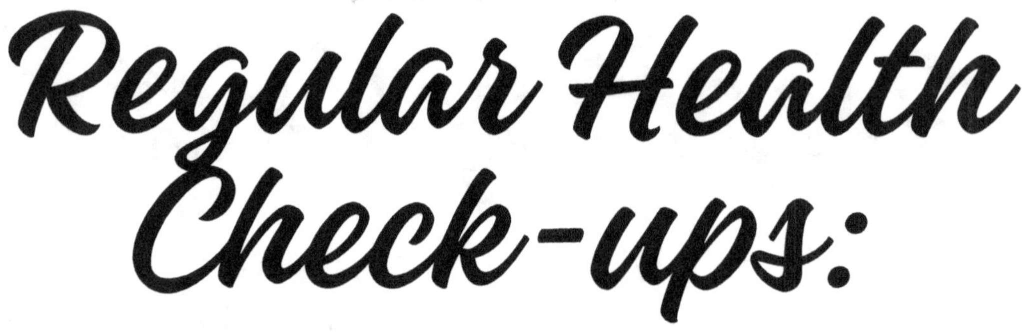

- Schedule regular check-ups with healthcare professionals to monitor and address any emerging health issues promptly.
- Discuss any concerns or symptoms with your healthcare provider to get appropriate guidance.

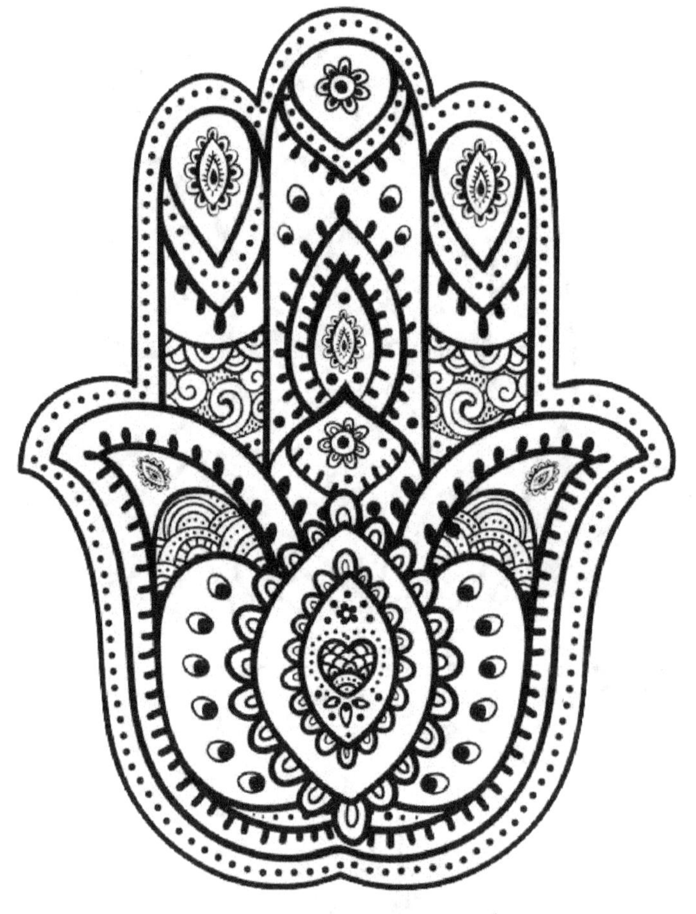

Adequate Sleep:

- Prioritize quality sleep to support overall well-being and the body's natural repair processes.
- Maintain a consistent sleep schedule and create a comfortable sleep environment.

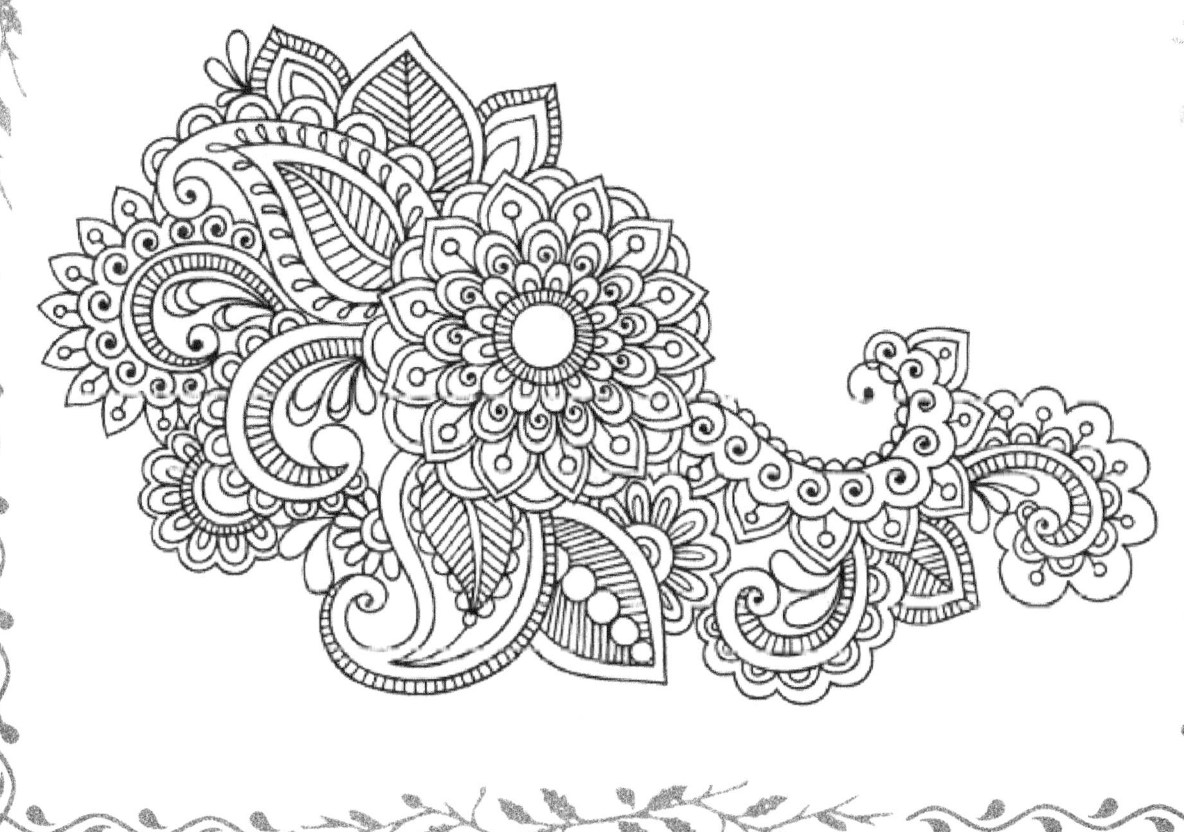

Manage Stress:

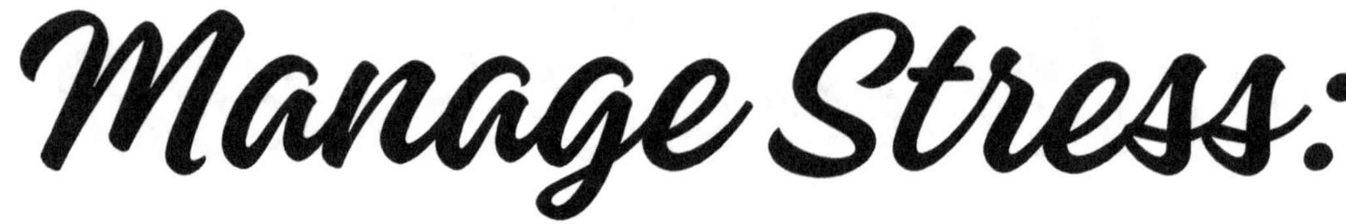

- Practice stress-reducing activities such as meditation, deep breathing, or yoga.
- Cultivate a support system of friends and family to share concerns and emotions.

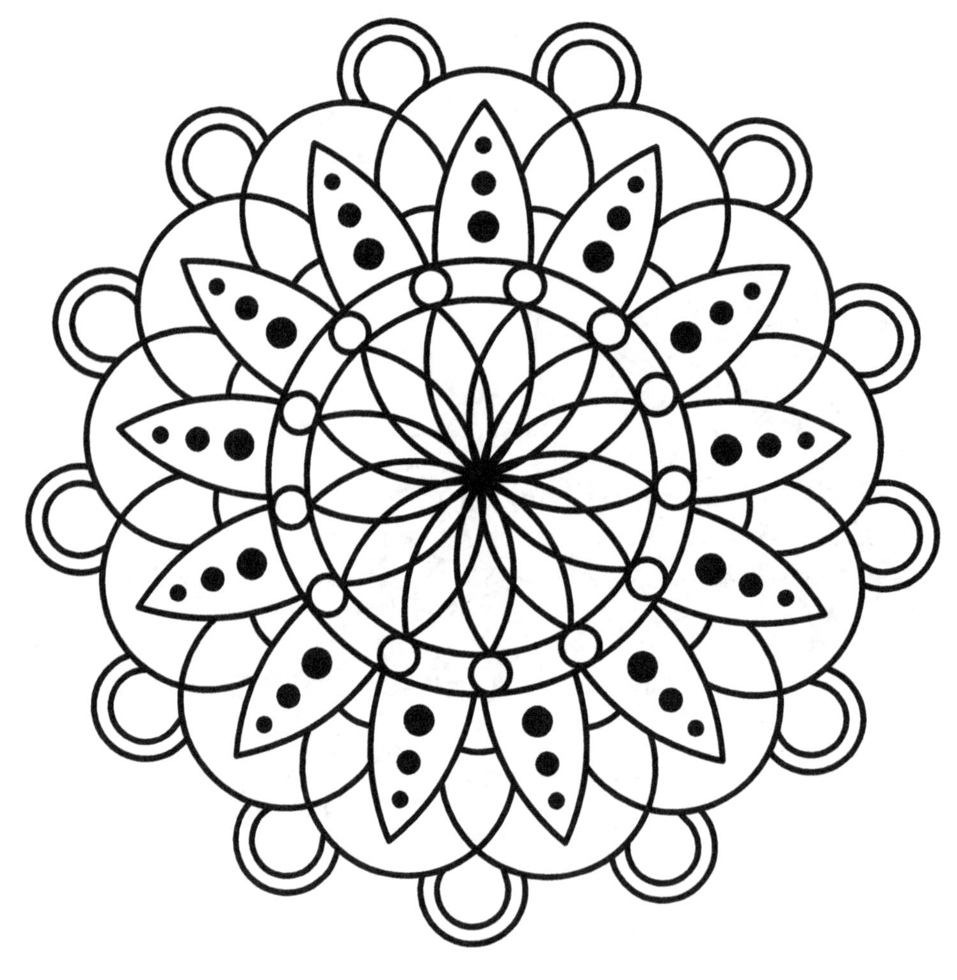

Joint Health:

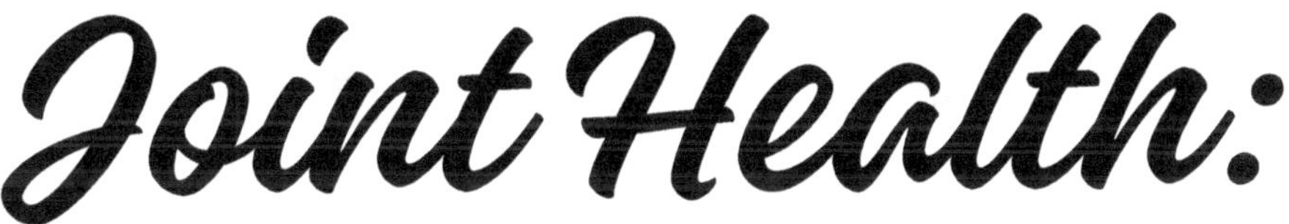

- Take steps to protect joint health by maintaining a healthy weight and incorporating joint-friendly exercises.
- Consider supplements like glucosamine and chondroitin, but consult with a healthcare professional first.

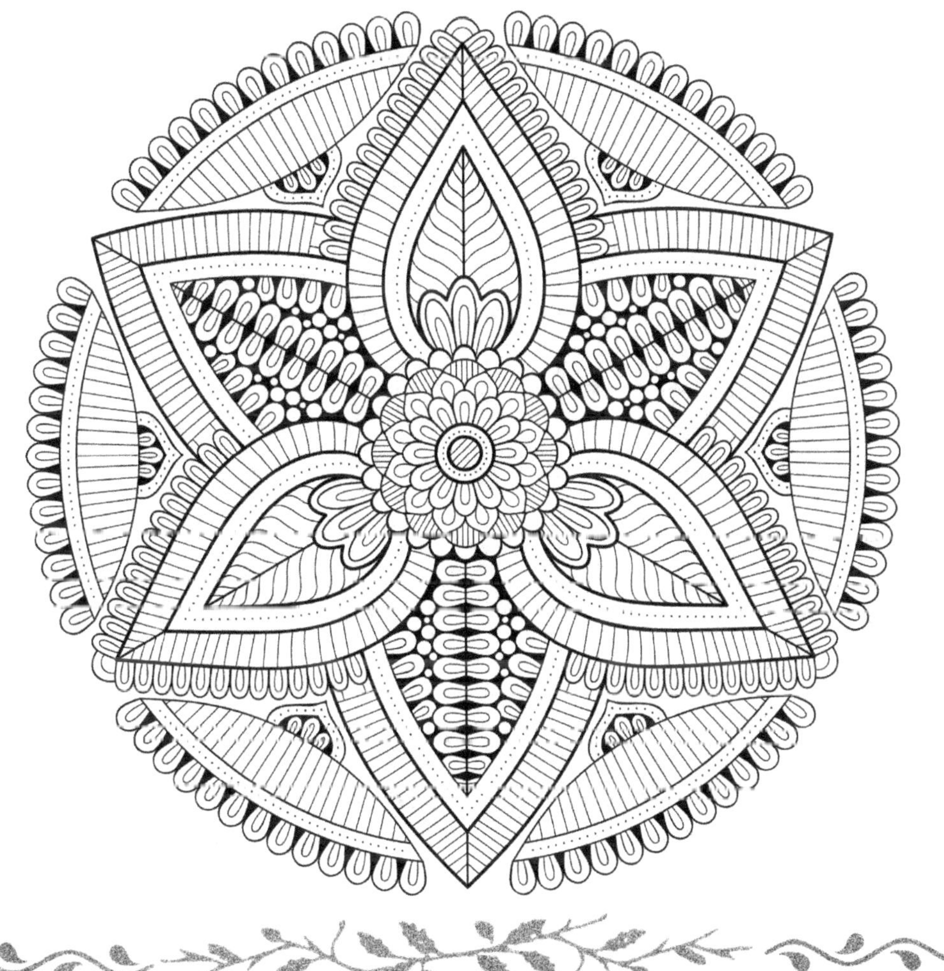

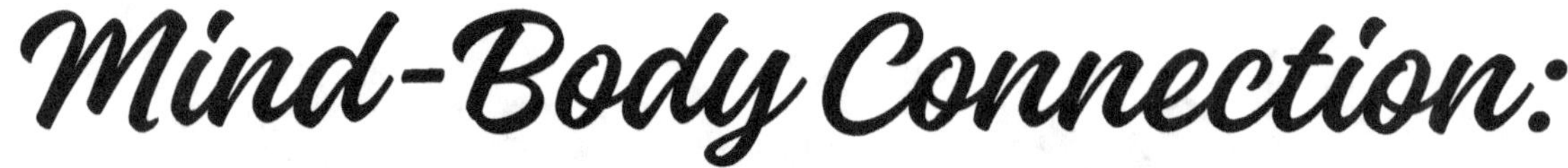

Mind-Body Connection:

- Engage in activities that promote mental well-being, such as mindfulness, meditation, or hobbies that bring joy.
- Stay mentally active through puzzles, reading, or learning new skills to stimulate cognitive function.

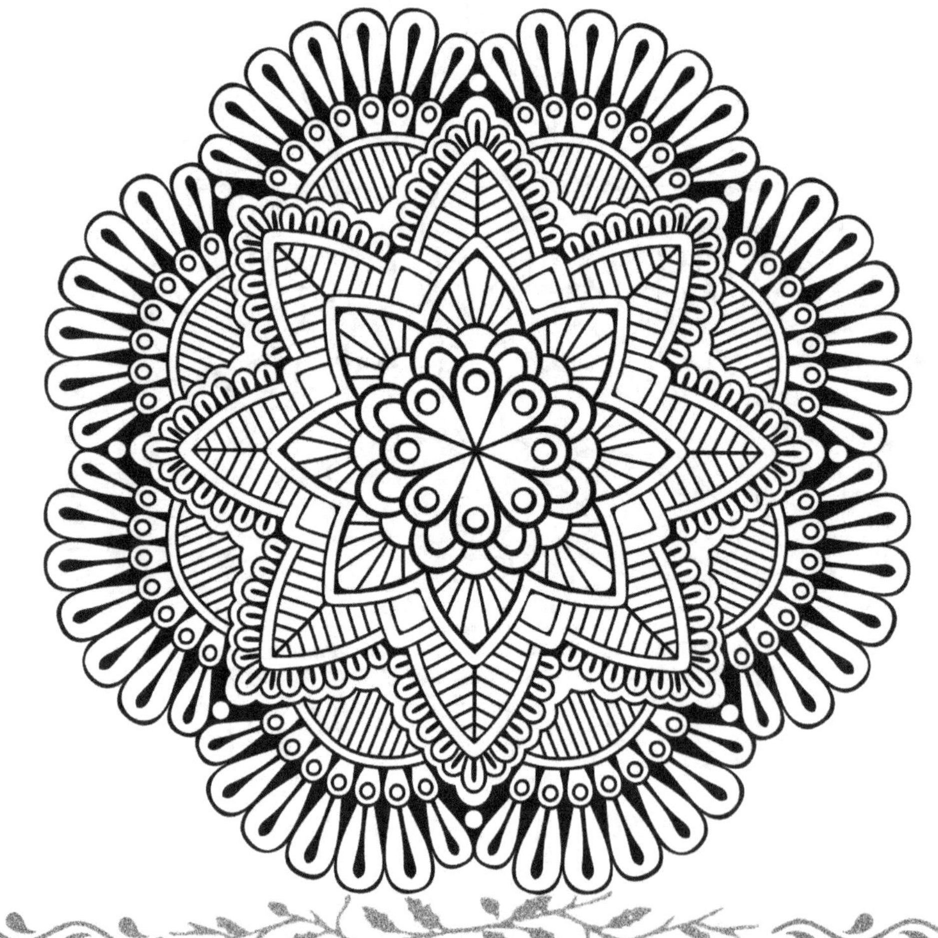

Stay Socially Connected:

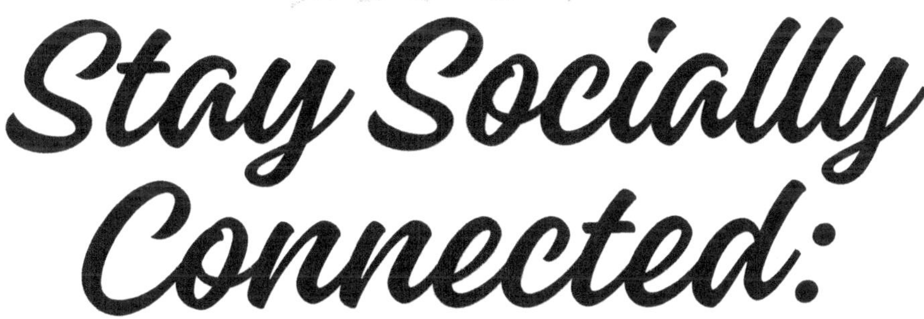

- Maintain social connections to prevent isolation, as social engagement is crucial for mental and emotional health.
- Join clubs, volunteer, or participate in community events to stay connected.

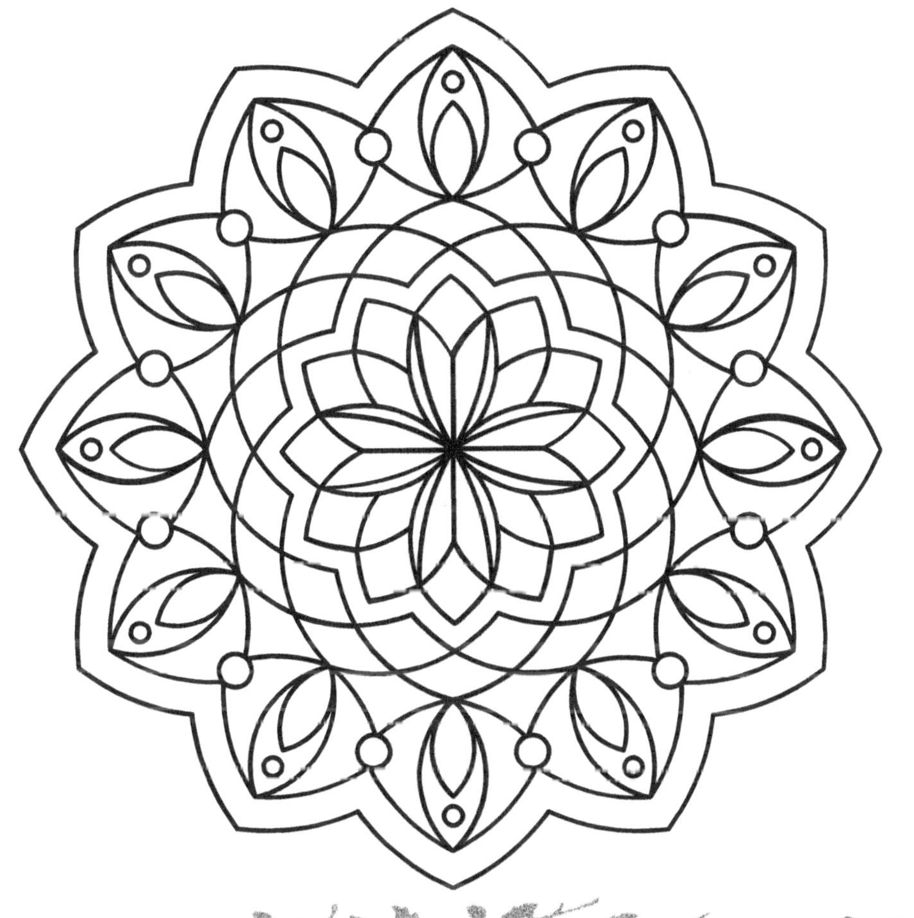

Adaptability:

- Be open to adapting your lifestyle to accommodate physical changes. This may involve using assistive devices or making modifications to your living space.
- Seek professional advice on mobility aids or modifications that can enhance safety and independence.

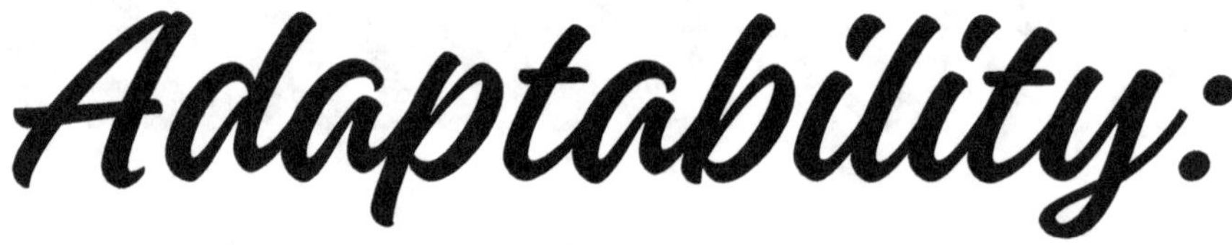

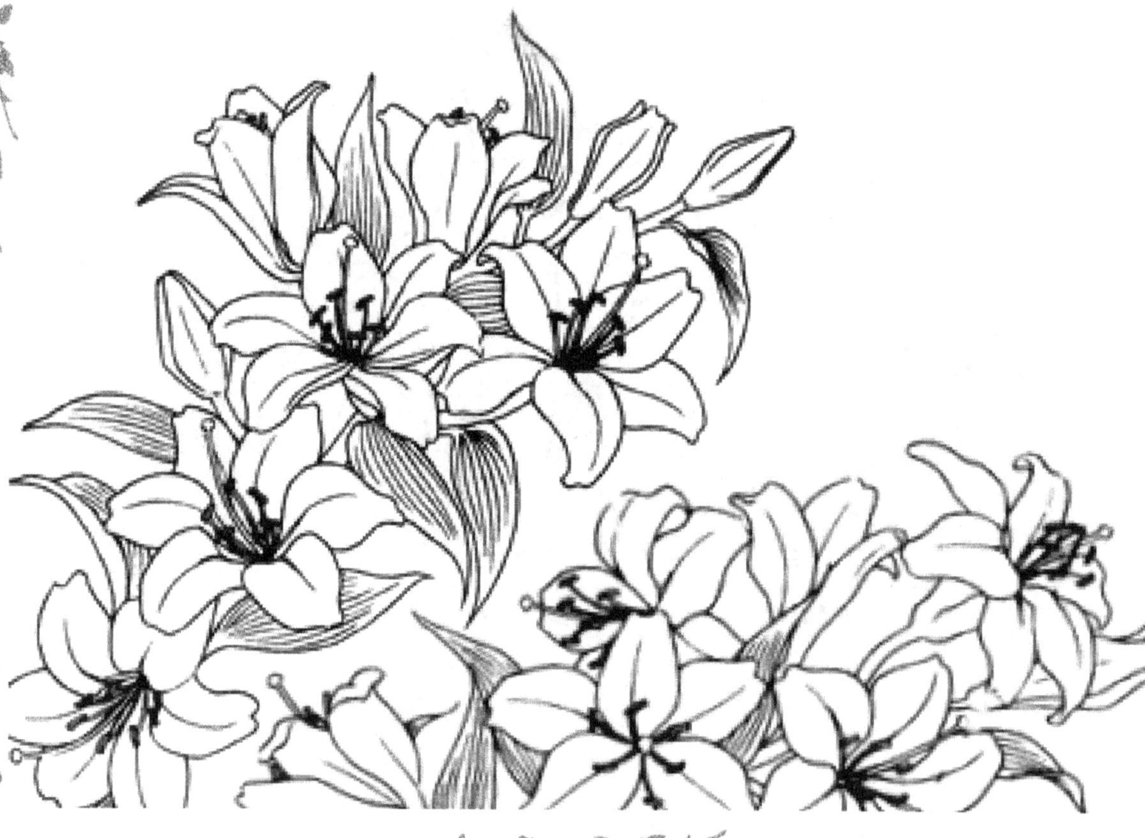

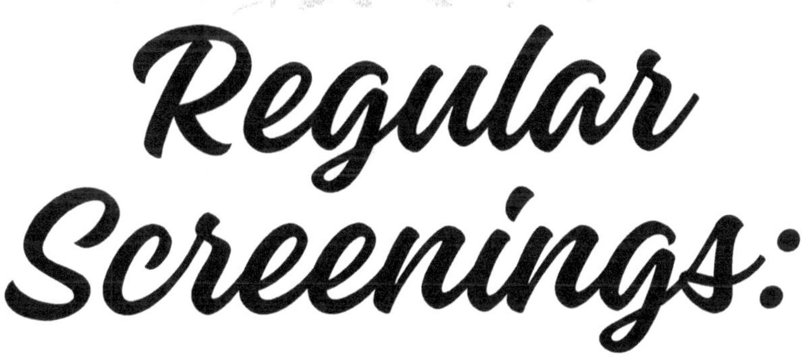

Regular Screenings:

- Participate in age-appropriate screenings for conditions such as osteoporosis, diabetes, and cardiovascular diseases.
- Early detection and management can significantly impact outcomes.
-

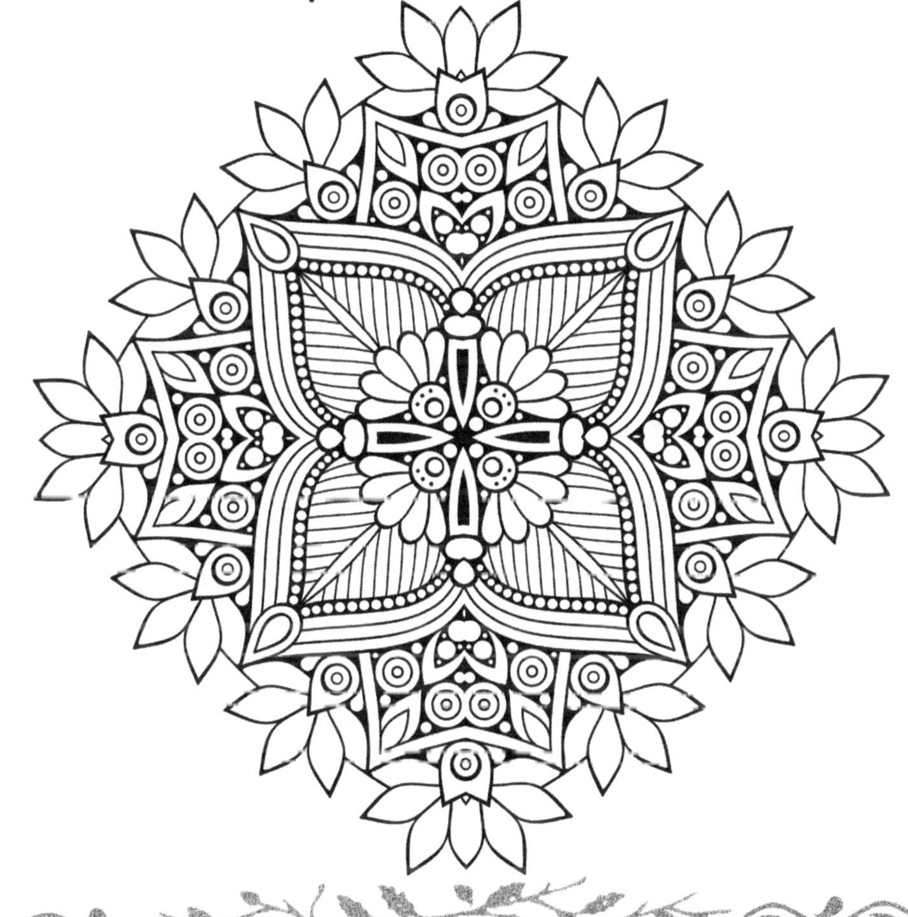

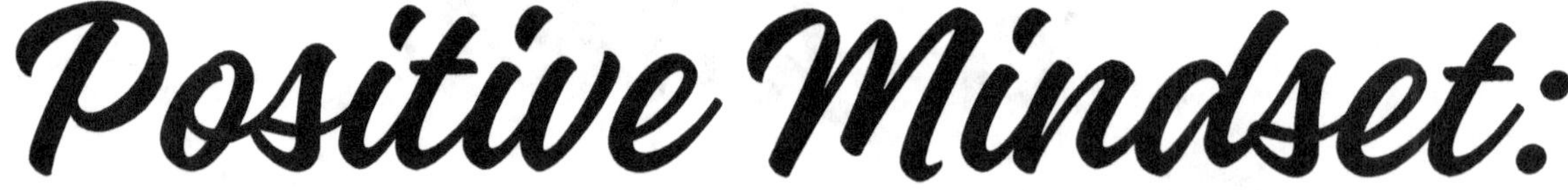

Positive Mindset:

- Cultivate a positive attitude toward aging. Embrace the wisdom and experience that come with getting older.
- Focus on what you can control and find fulfillment in new experiences and relationships.
-

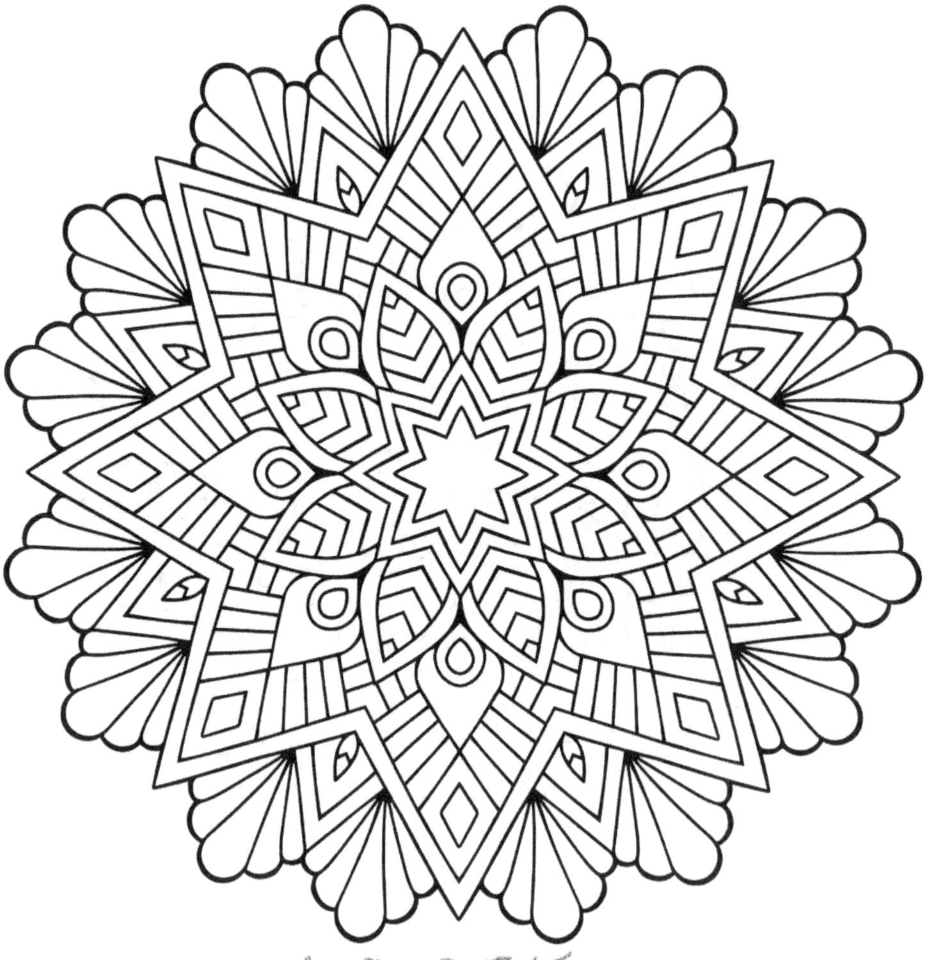

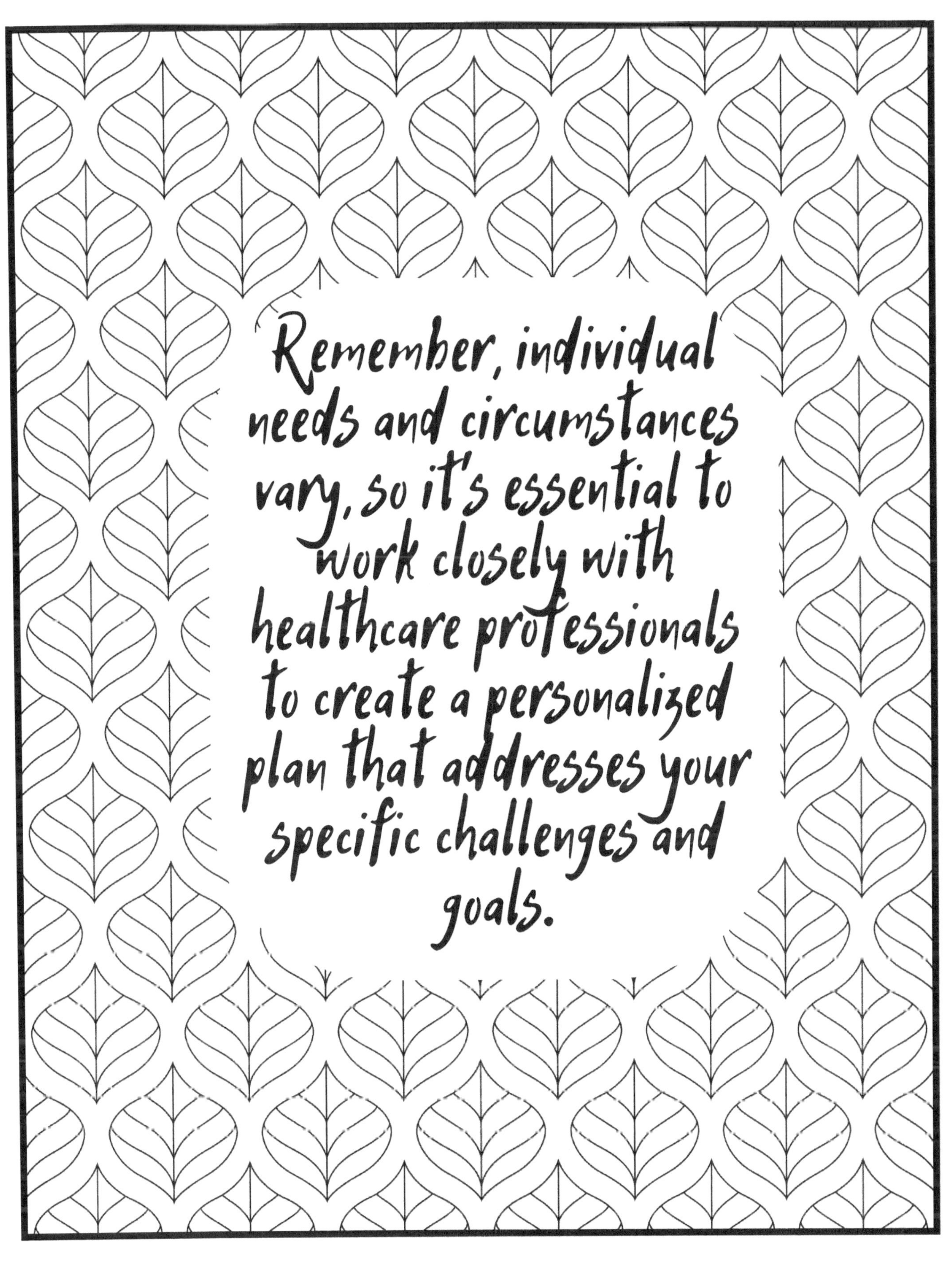

Remember, individual needs and circumstances vary, so it's essential to work closely with healthcare professionals to create a personalized plan that addresses your specific challenges and goals.

Hygiene and Self-Care:

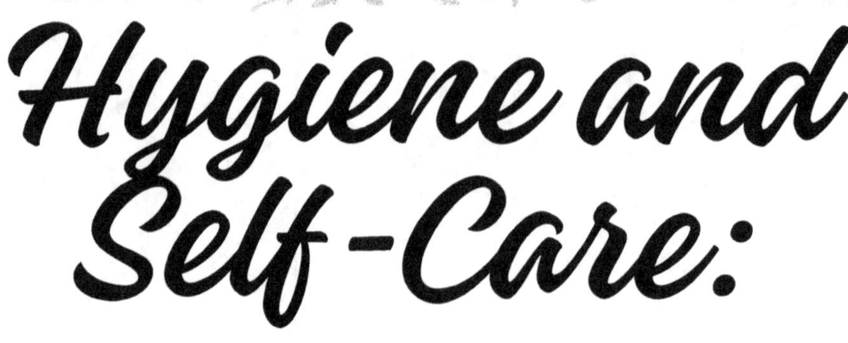

- Prioritize personal hygiene and self-care routines to maintain overall health and well-being.
- Regular grooming practices can contribute to a positive self-image and boost confidence.

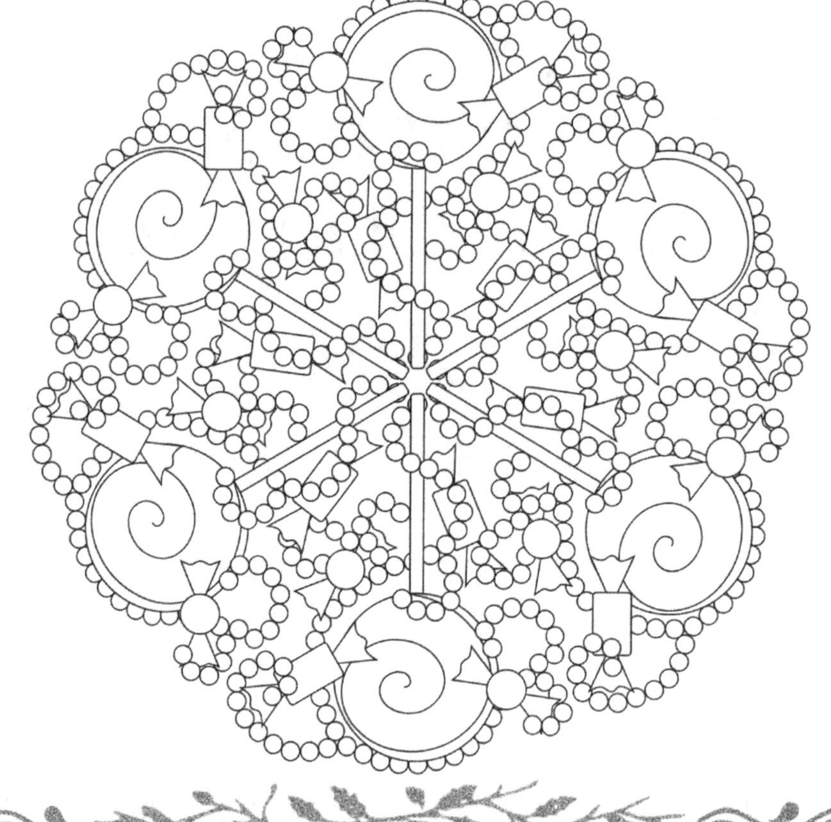

Vision and Hearing Health:

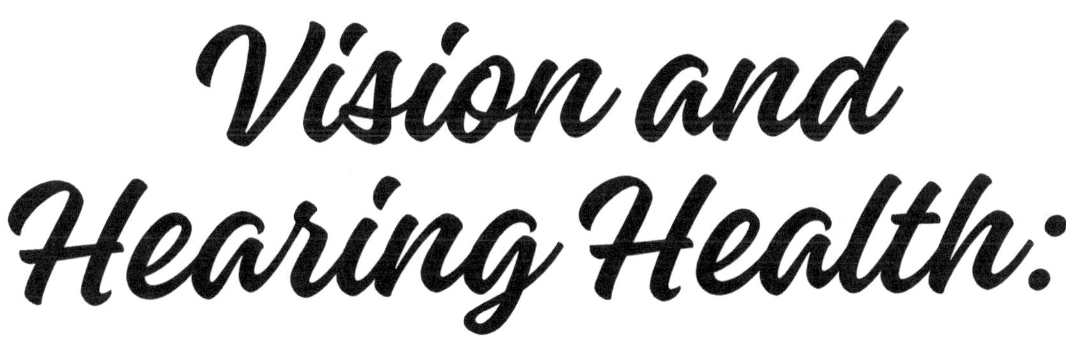

- Schedule regular eye and ear check-ups to address changes in vision and hearing.
- Use corrective lenses or hearing aids as recommended to enhance daily functioning.

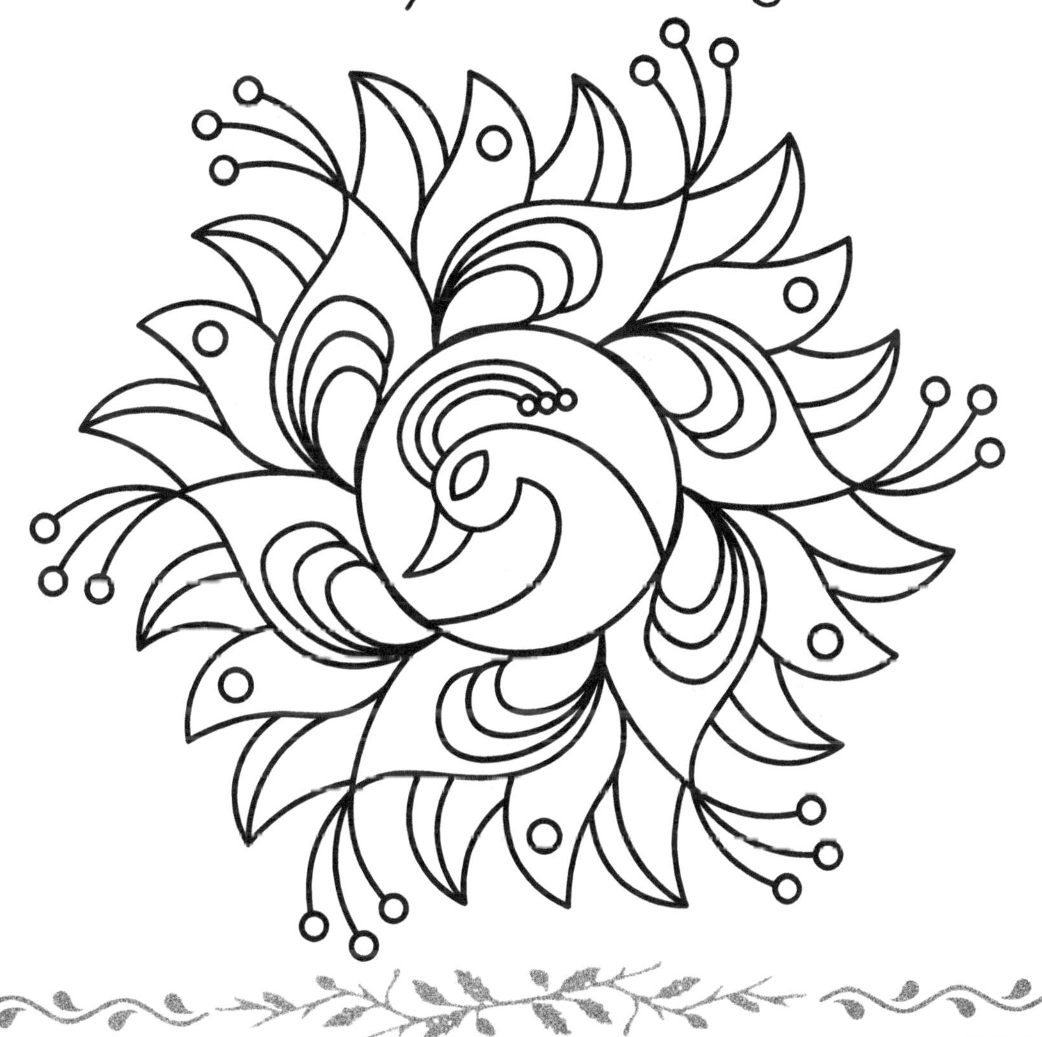

Balance and Fall Prevention:

- Practice exercises that improve balance and stability, such as tai chi or yoga.
- Ensure your living space is free of hazards, and consider installing handrails and grab bars to reduce the risk of falls.

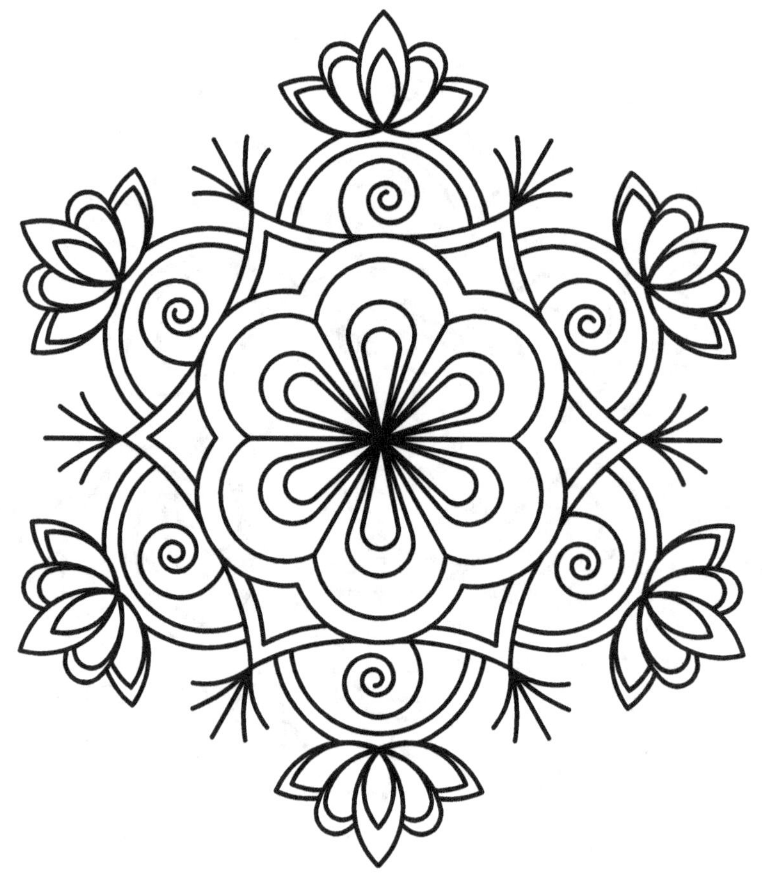

Medication Management:

- Keep an updated list of medications, including dosages and schedules.
- Communicate regularly with your healthcare provider to discuss any side effects or potential interactions.

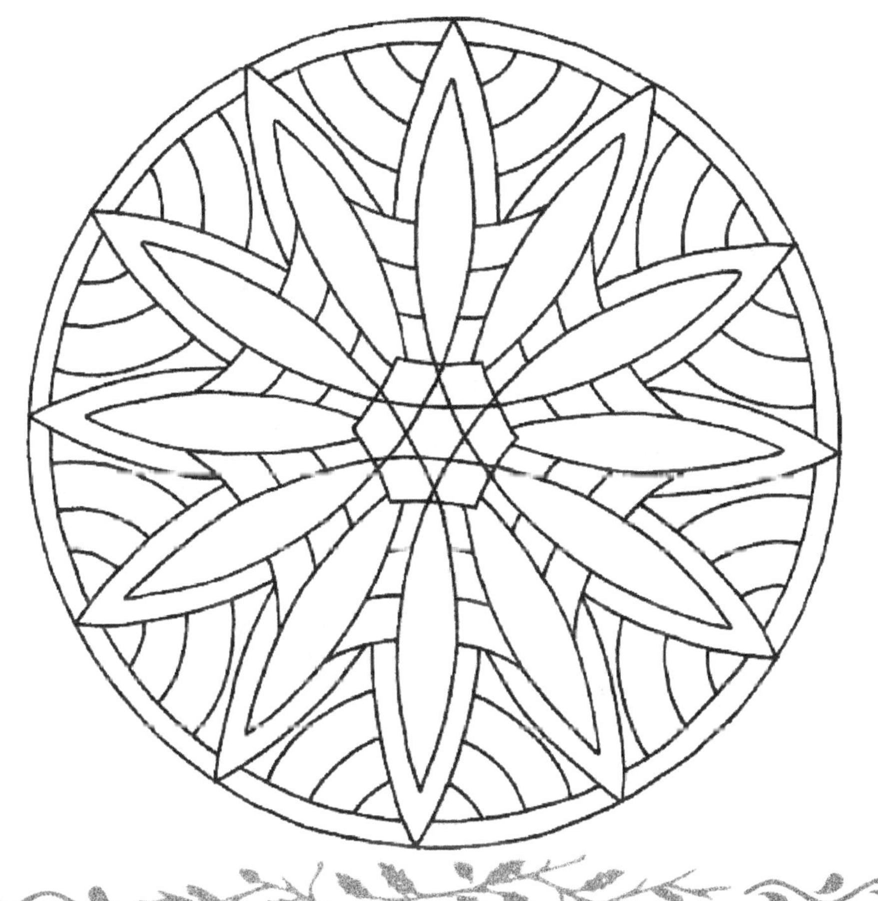

Pain Management:

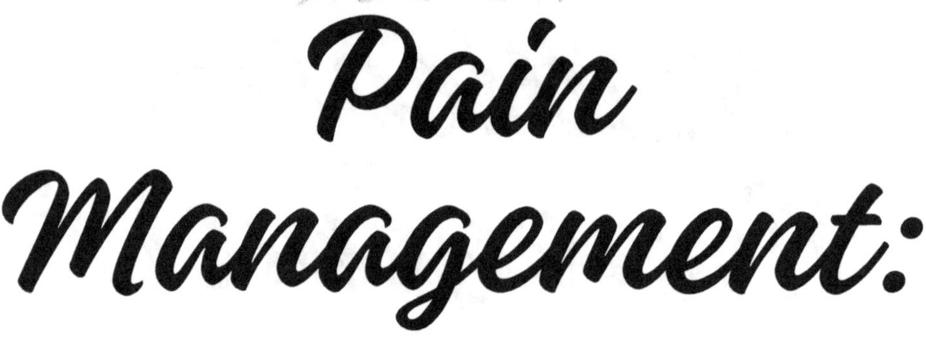

- Seek medical advice for managing chronic pain through a combination of medication, physical therapy, and alternative therapies.
- Stay active, as appropriate, to promote joint flexibility and reduce stiffness.

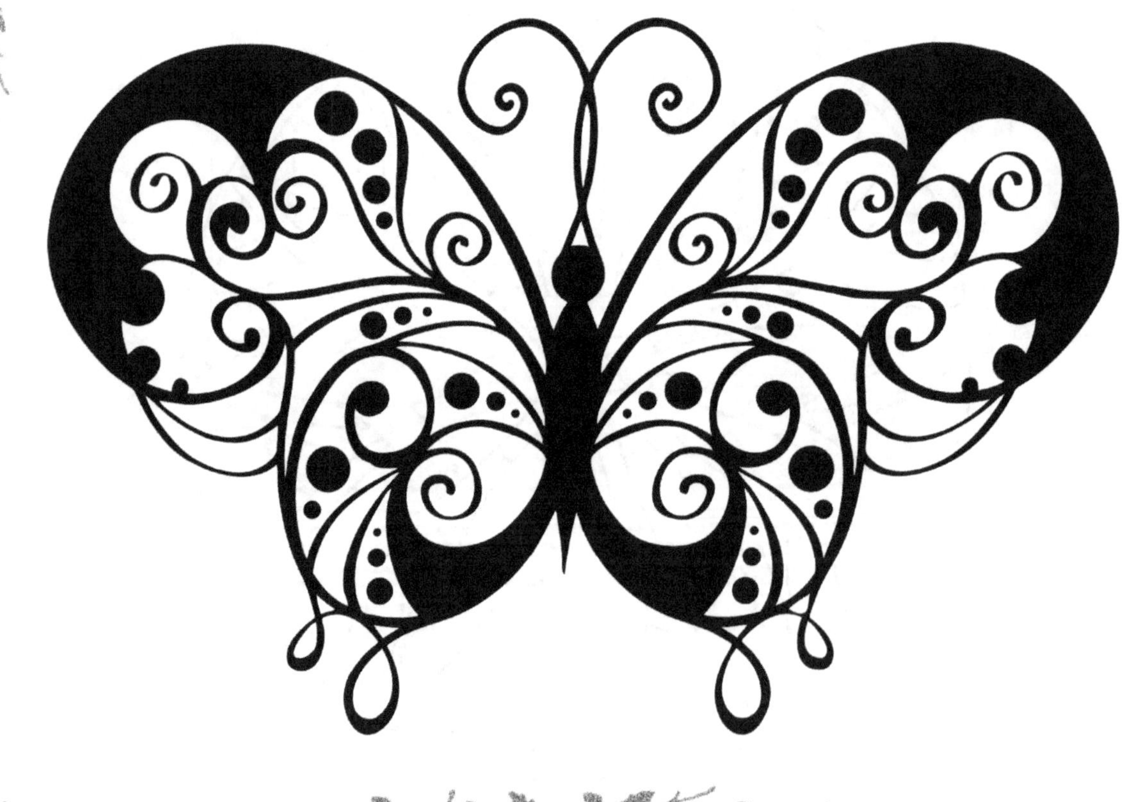

Technology for Assistance:

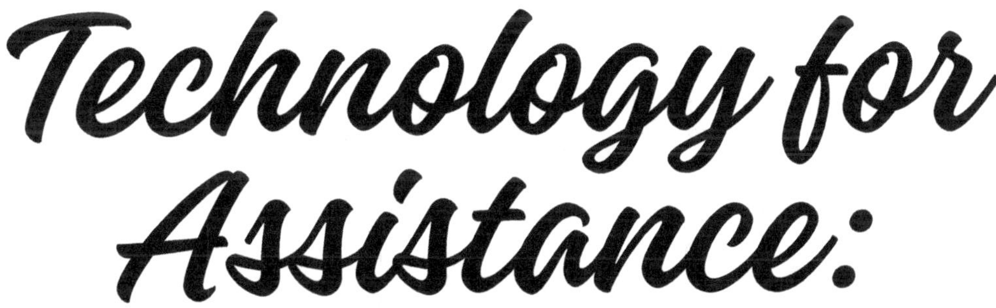

- Explore technology options that can assist in daily activities, such as medication reminders, fitness apps, and communication tools.
- Stay informed about new technologies designed to enhance the lives of older adults.

Financial Planning:

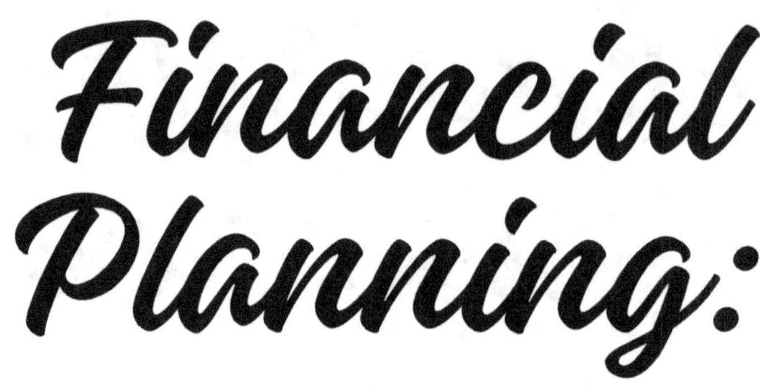

- Plan for your financial future, considering healthcare costs, insurance coverage, and potential long-term care needs.
- Consult with a financial advisor to create a sustainable plan for your retirement years.

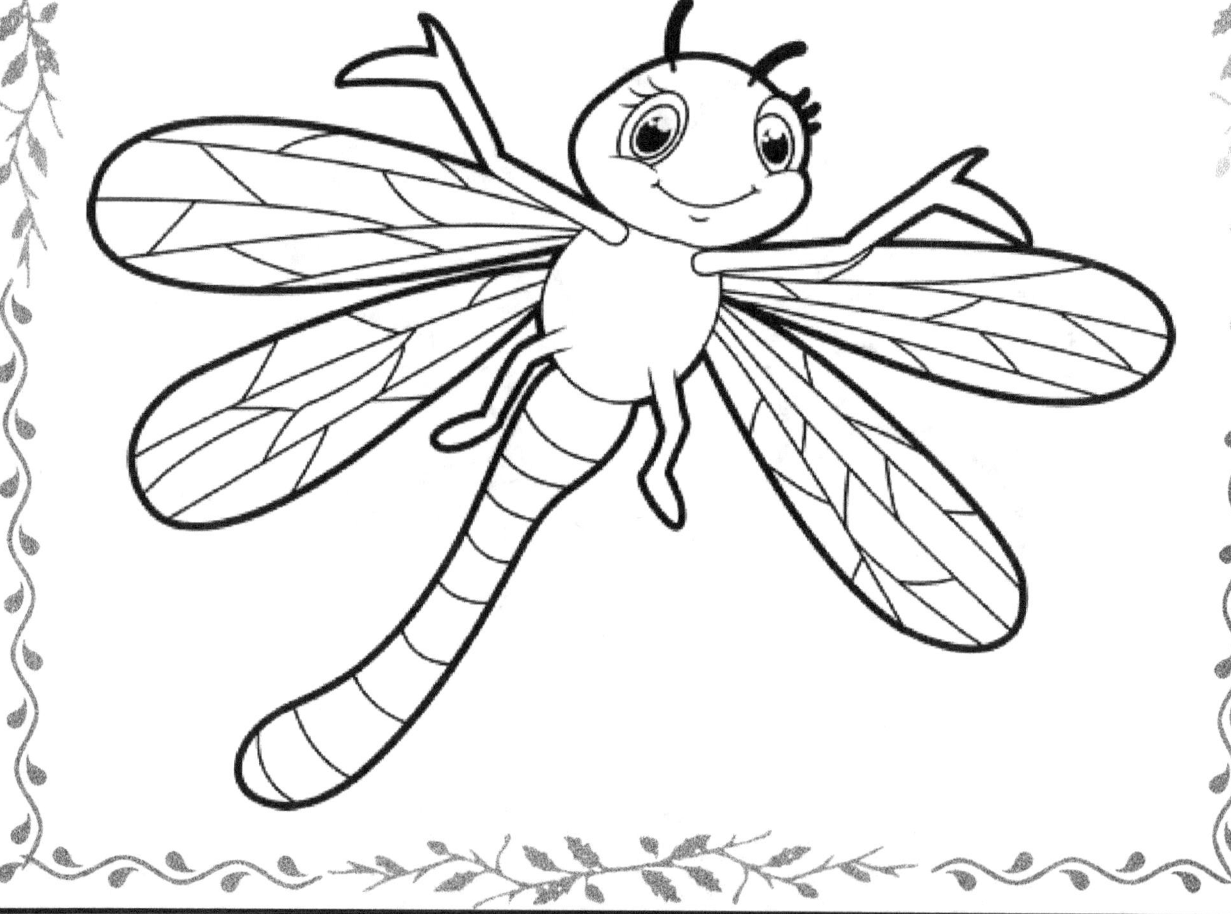

Continual Learning:

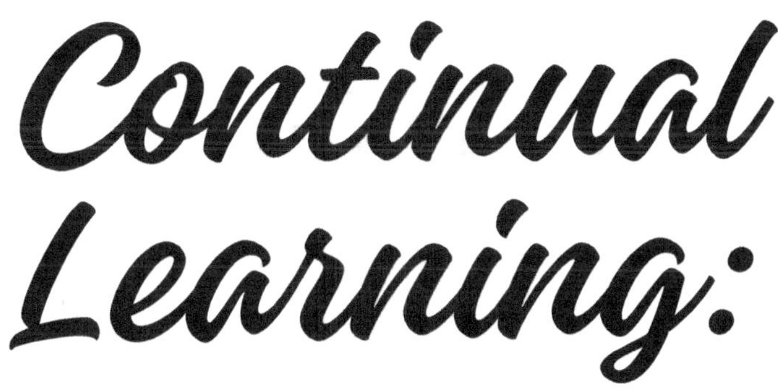

- Stay intellectually engaged by pursuing hobbies, taking classes, or learning new skills.
- Engaging in lifelong learning not only stimulates the mind but also provides a sense of accomplishment.

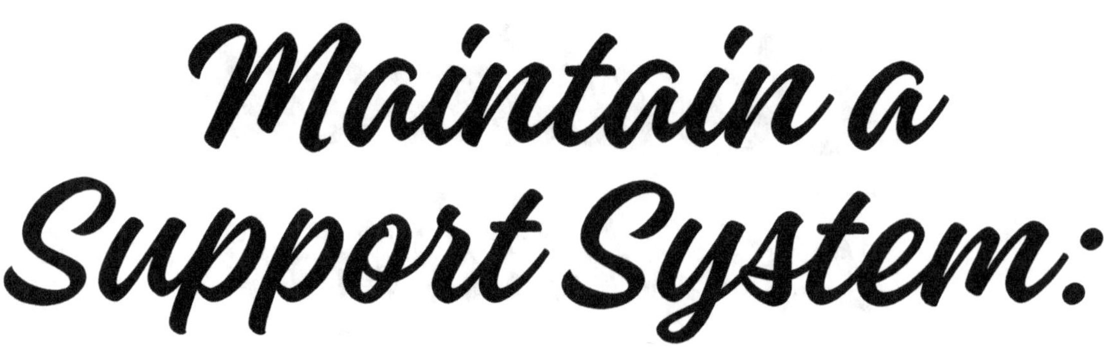

Maintain a Support System:

- Nurture relationships with family and friends who provide emotional support and companionship.
- Join social groups or clubs that share your interests, fostering a sense of community.

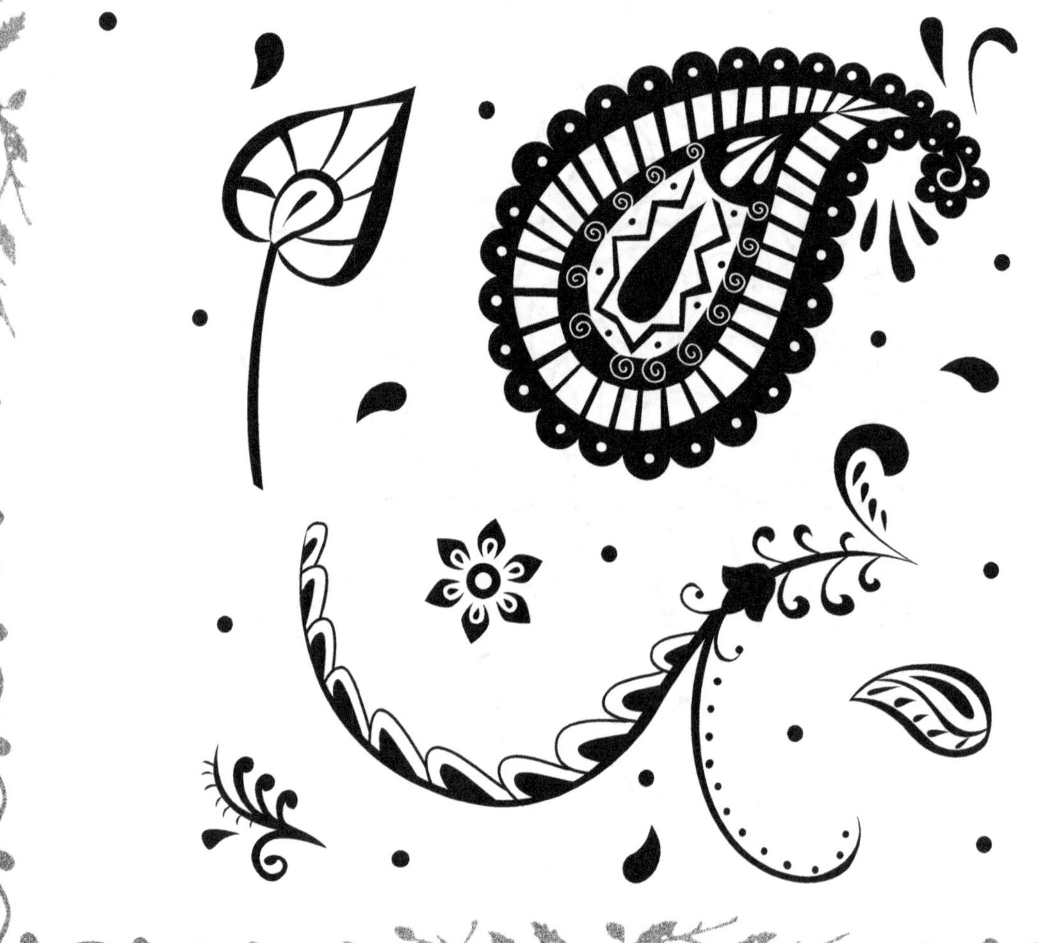

Explore Therapeutic Options:

- Consider complementary therapies such as massage, acupuncture, or physical therapy to address specific health concerns.
- Consult with healthcare professionals to ensure these therapies align with your overall wellness plan.

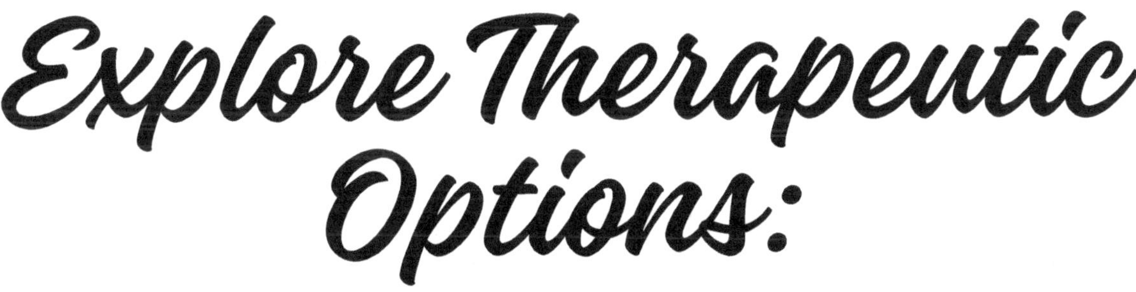

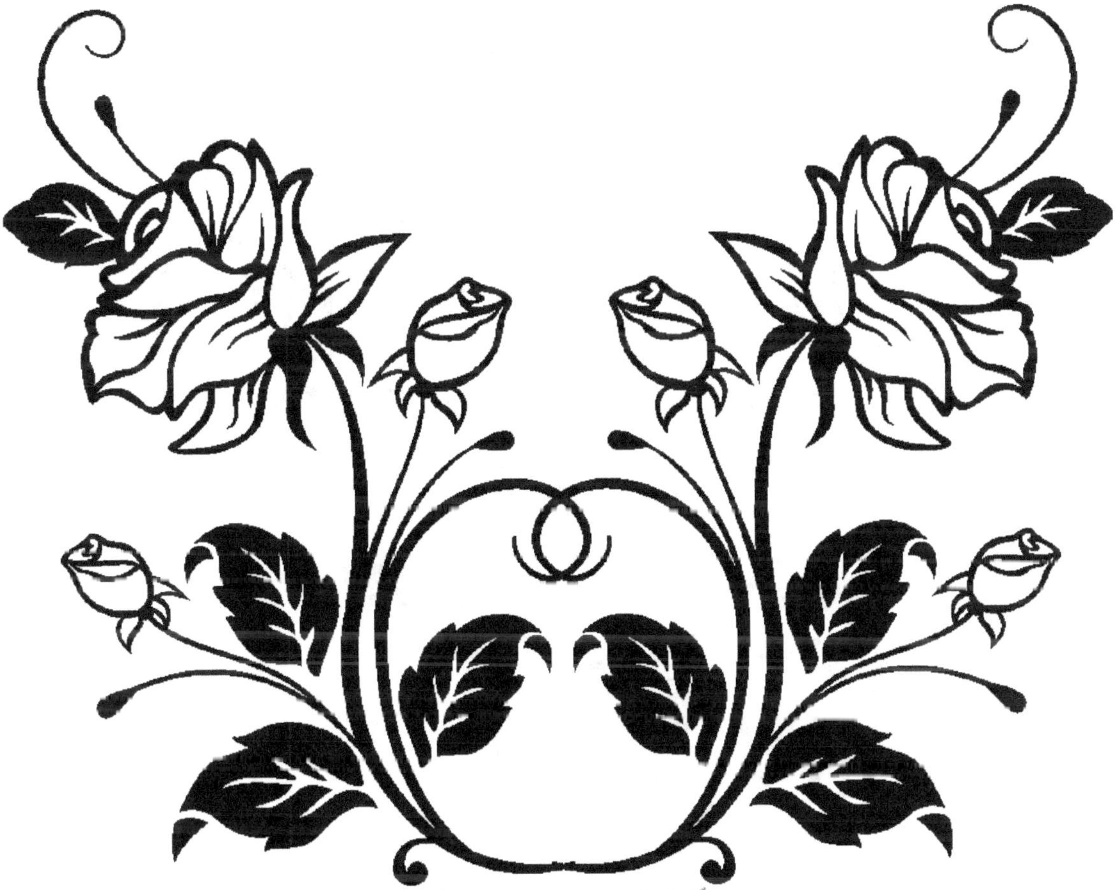

Plan for Transitions:

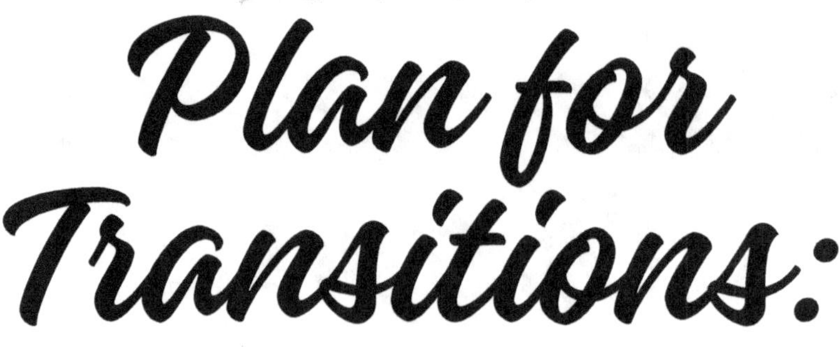

- Be proactive in planning for potential transitions in living arrangements or care needs.
- Communicate your preferences with loved ones and explore options for home modifications or assisted living if needed.

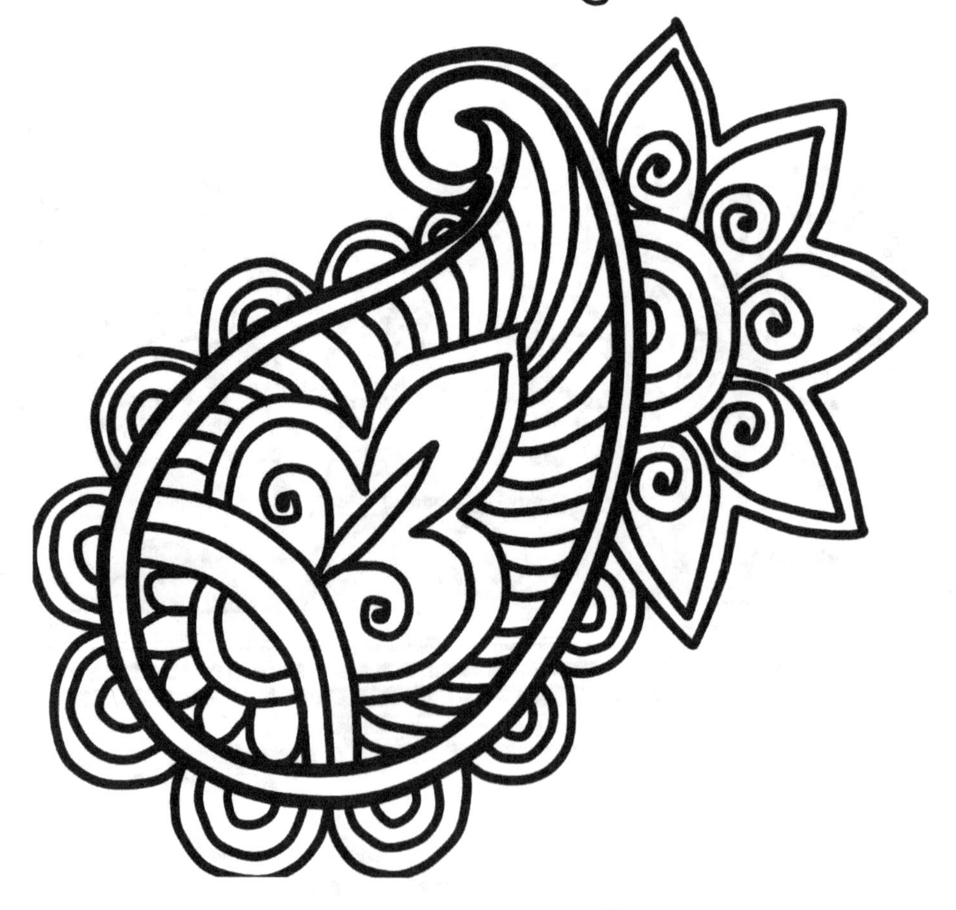

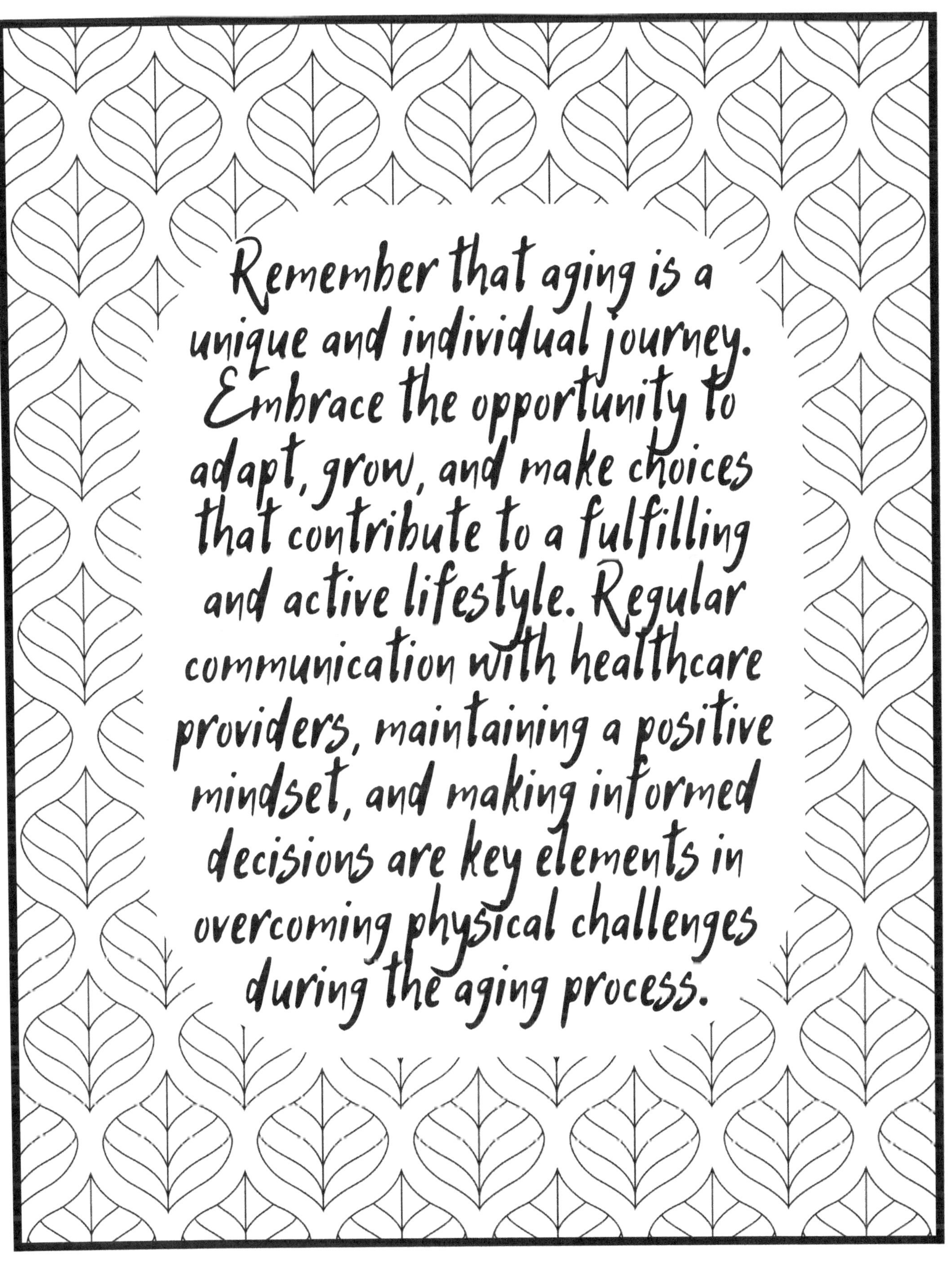

Remember that aging is a unique and individual journey. Embrace the opportunity to adapt, grow, and make choices that contribute to a fulfilling and active lifestyle. Regular communication with healthcare providers, maintaining a positive mindset, and making informed decisions are key elements in overcoming physical challenges during the aging process.

Cultivate a Sense of Purpose:

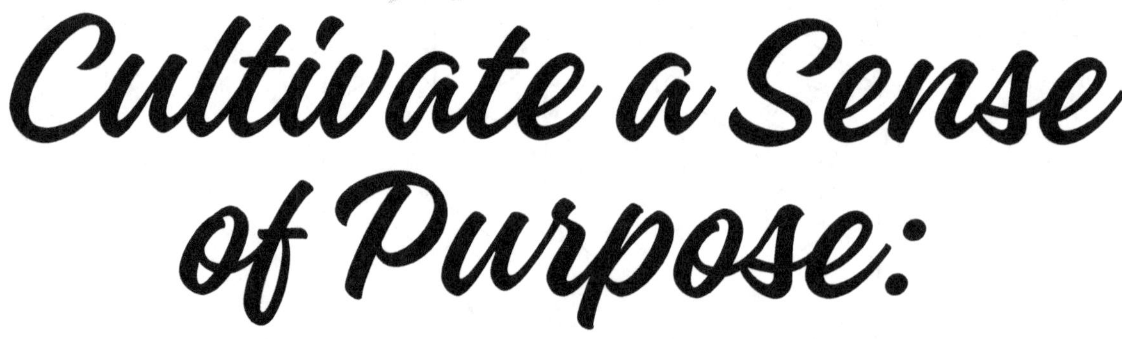

- Stay involved in activities that bring meaning and purpose to your life, whether through volunteering, mentoring, or pursuing personal passions.
- Having a sense of purpose can positively impact mental and emotional well-being.

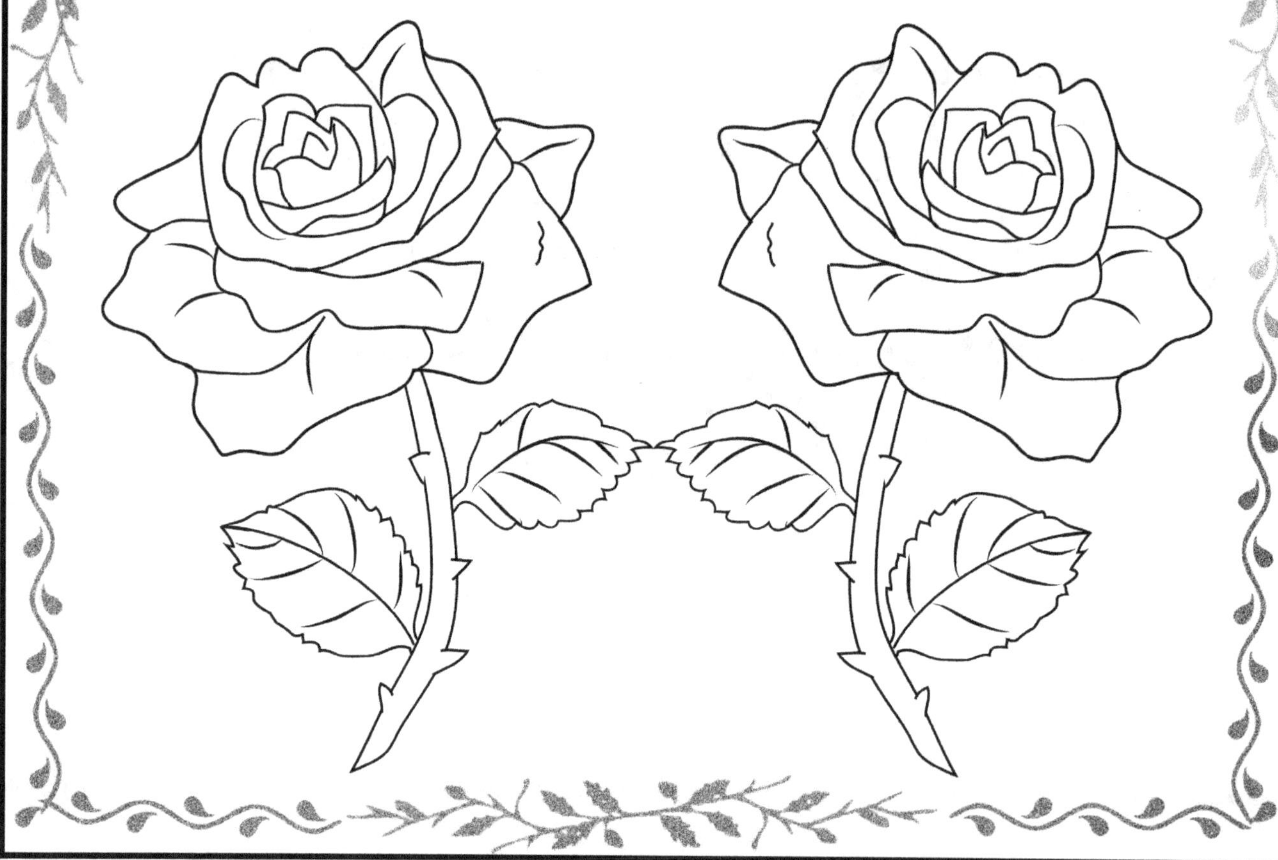

Sun Protection:

- Protect your skin from the sun by using sunscreen, wearing protective clothing, and seeking shade.
- Regularly check your skin for any unusual moles or changes and consult a dermatologist if needed.

Stay Informed About Health Advances:

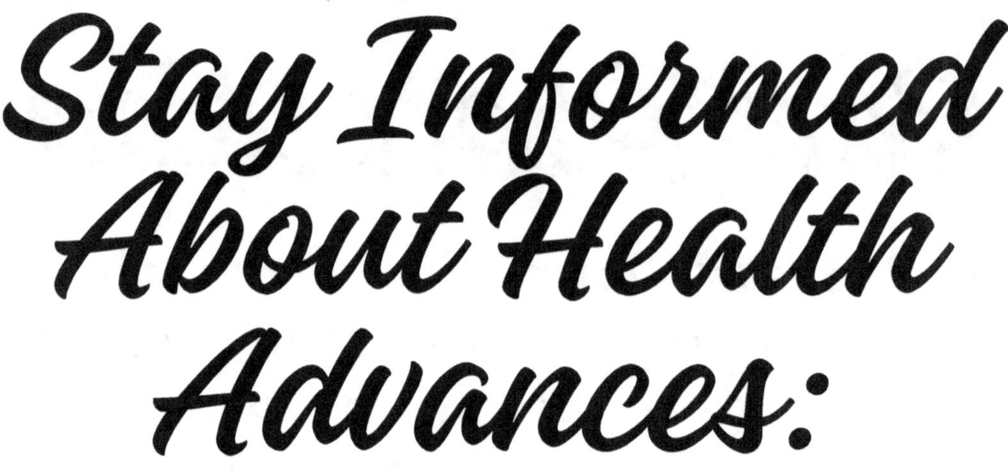

- Stay updated on medical research and advancements in healthcare that may offer new solutions or treatments.
- Discuss any potential innovations with your healthcare provider to see if they align with your health goals.

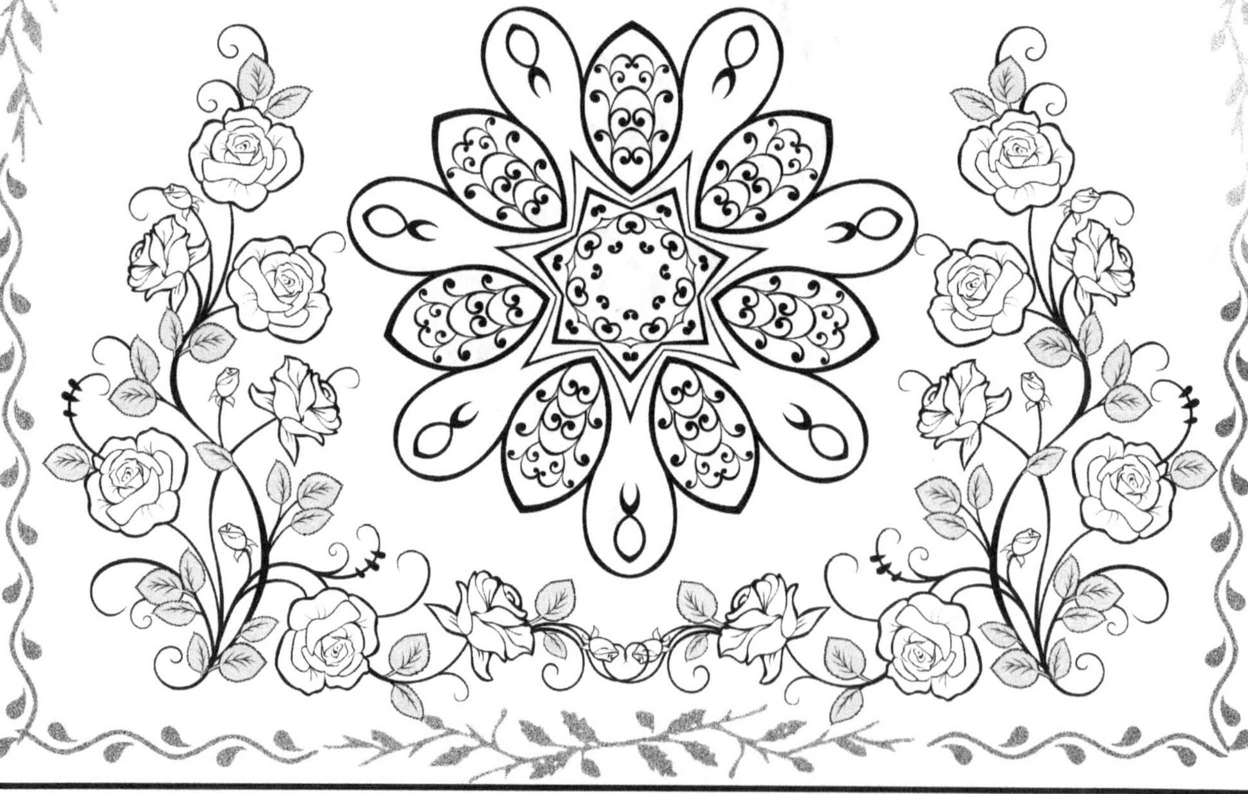

Embrace Technology for Mental Stimulation:

- Use technology to engage in mental exercises and games that stimulate cognitive function.
- Stay connected with friends and family through video calls and social media to maintain a sense of community.

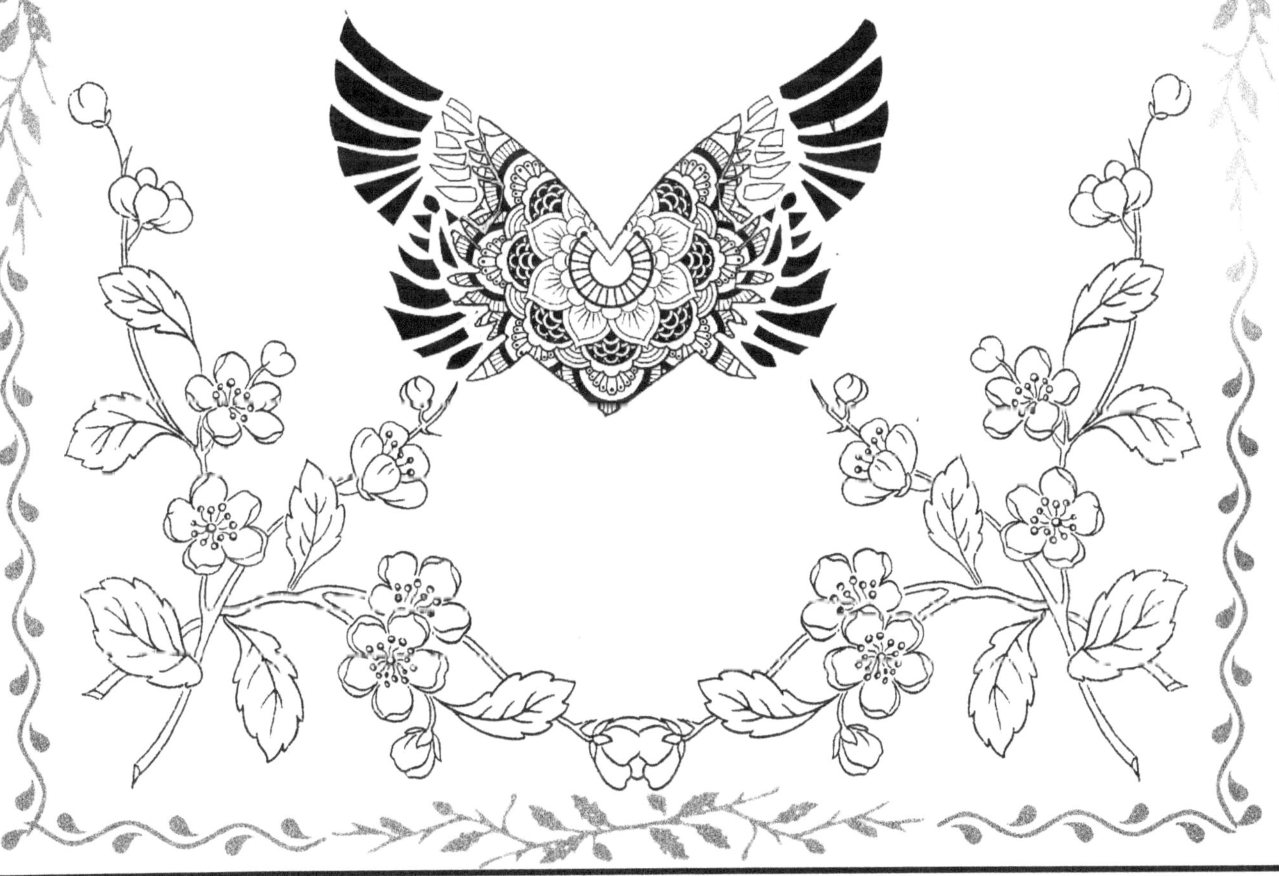

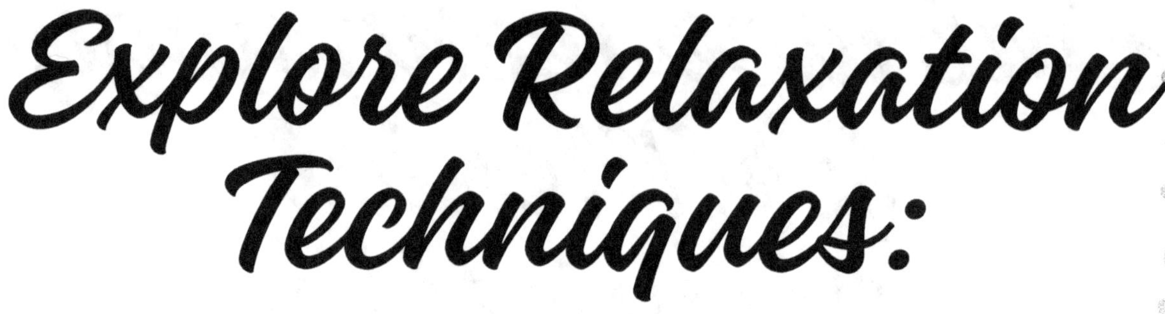

- Practice relaxation techniques such as progressive muscle relaxation or guided imagery to manage stress.
- Consider incorporating activities like gentle stretching or meditation into your daily routine.

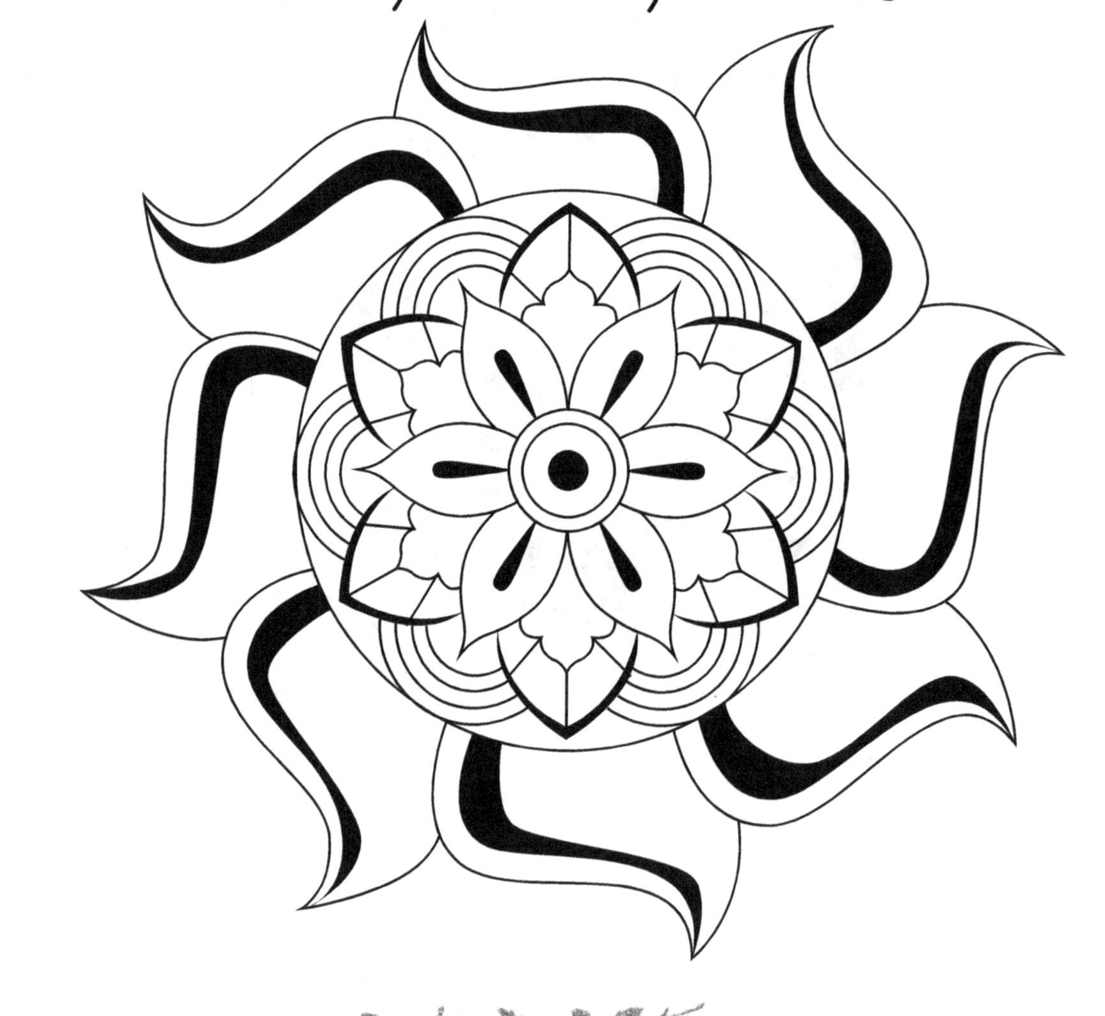

Plan for End-of-Life Care:

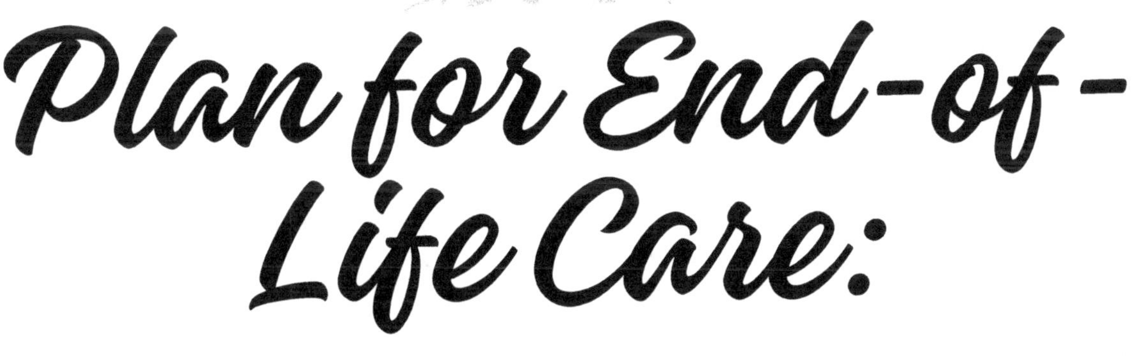

- Have open and honest conversations with loved ones about your preferences for end-of-life care.
- Consider creating advance directives and designating a healthcare proxy to ensure your wishes are respected.

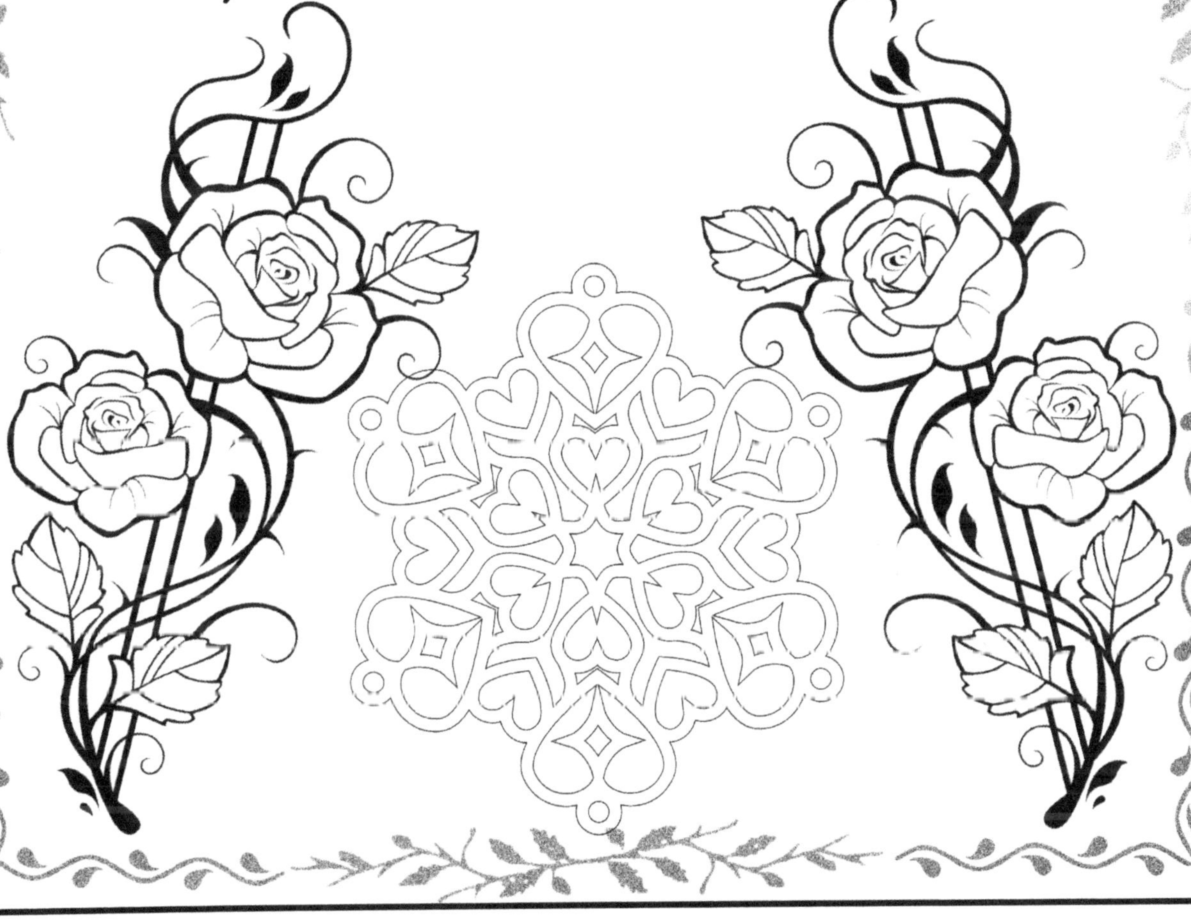

Engage in Brain-Boosting Activities:

- Challenge your brain with puzzles, crossword puzzles, Sudoku, or other mentally stimulating games.
- Learning new skills or taking up new hobbies can also contribute to cognitive health.

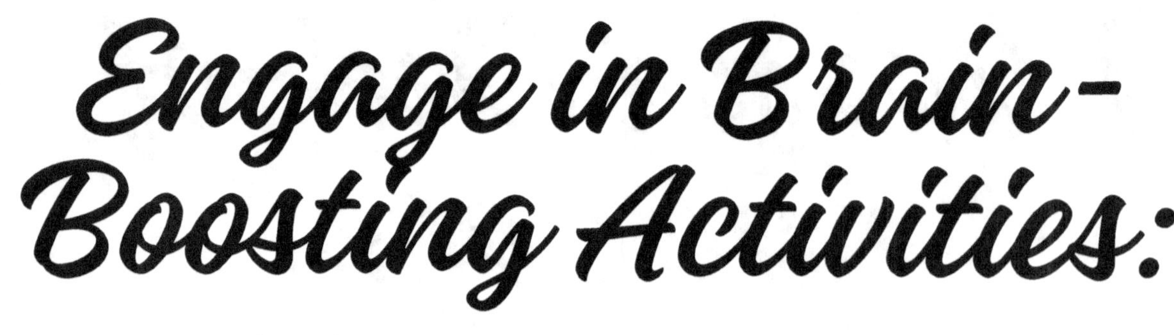

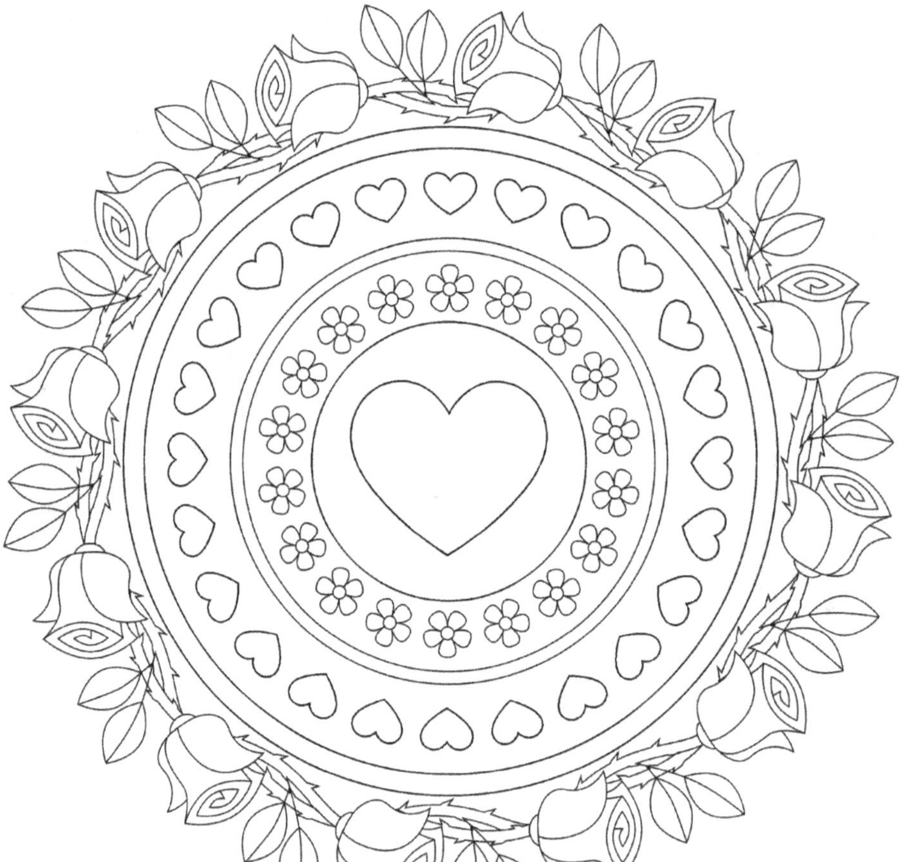

Adopt Healthy Habits Gradually:

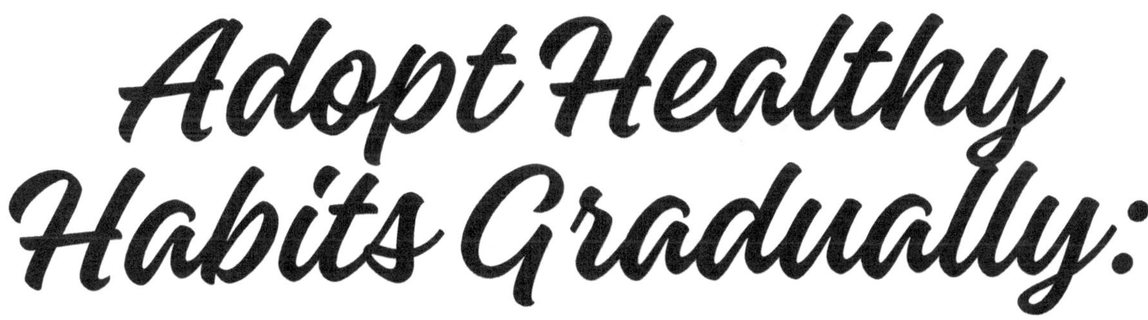

- If you're making significant lifestyle changes, consider implementing them gradually to allow for adjustment.
- Small, sustainable changes are often more effective and easier to maintain over the long term.

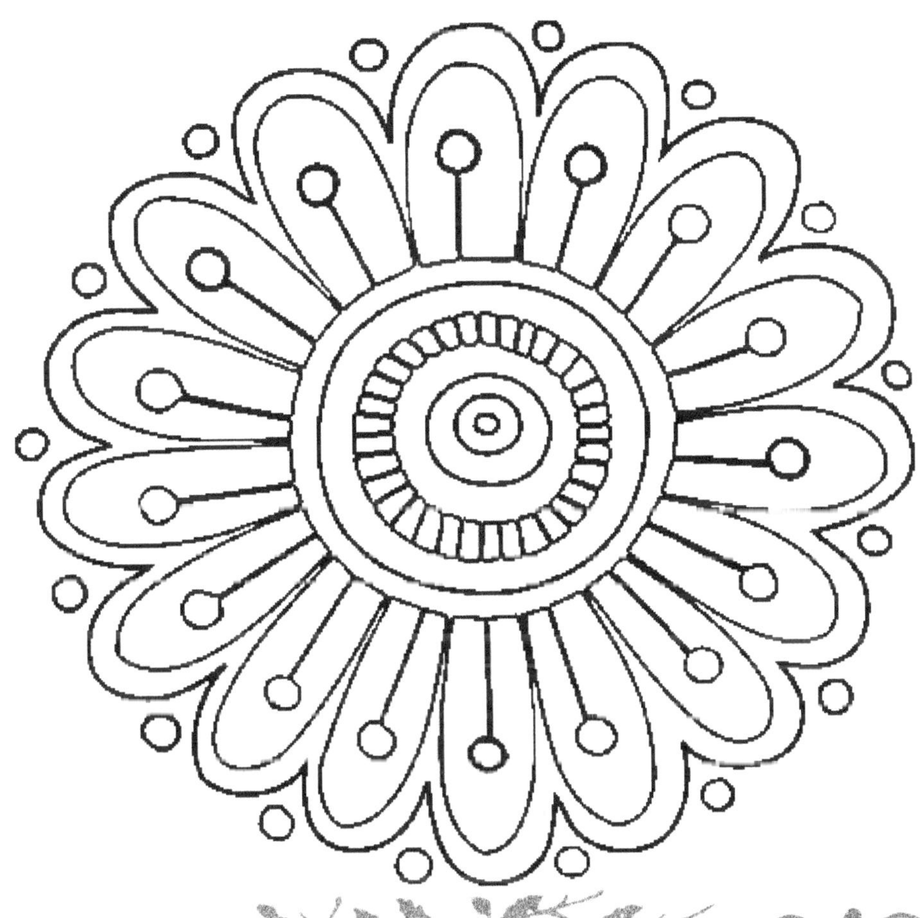

Celebrate Achievements:

- Acknowledge and celebrate milestones, no matter how small.
- Recognizing your achievements can boost self-esteem and motivation.

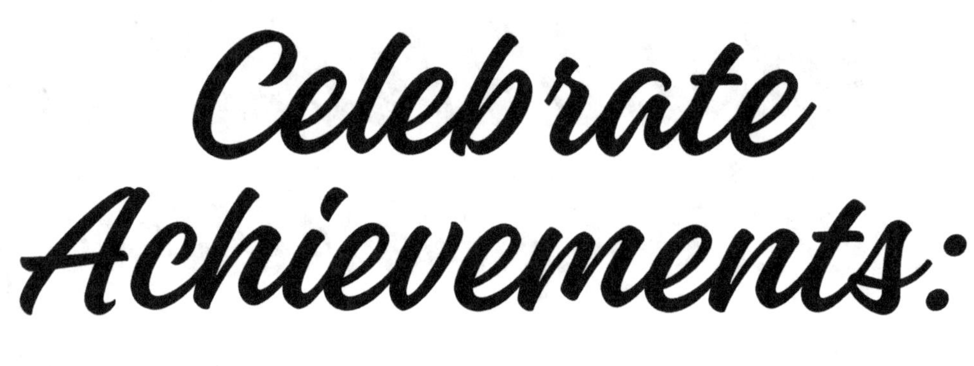

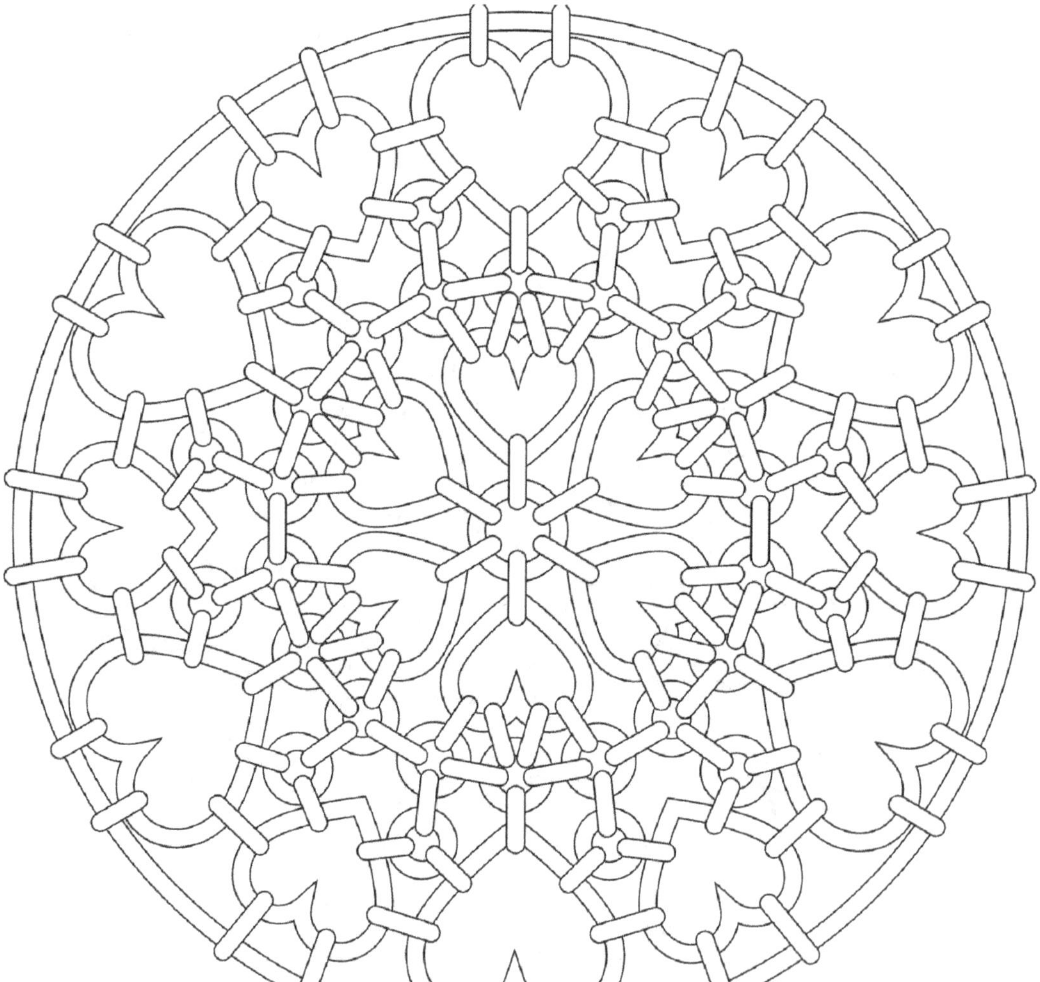

Maintain a Sense of Humor:

- Cultivate a sense of humor and find joy in everyday moments.
- Laughter has numerous health benefits, including stress reduction and improved mood.

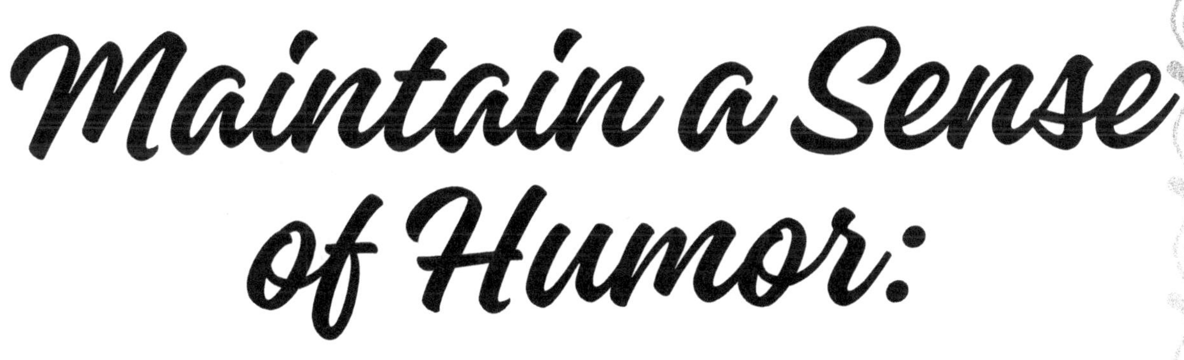

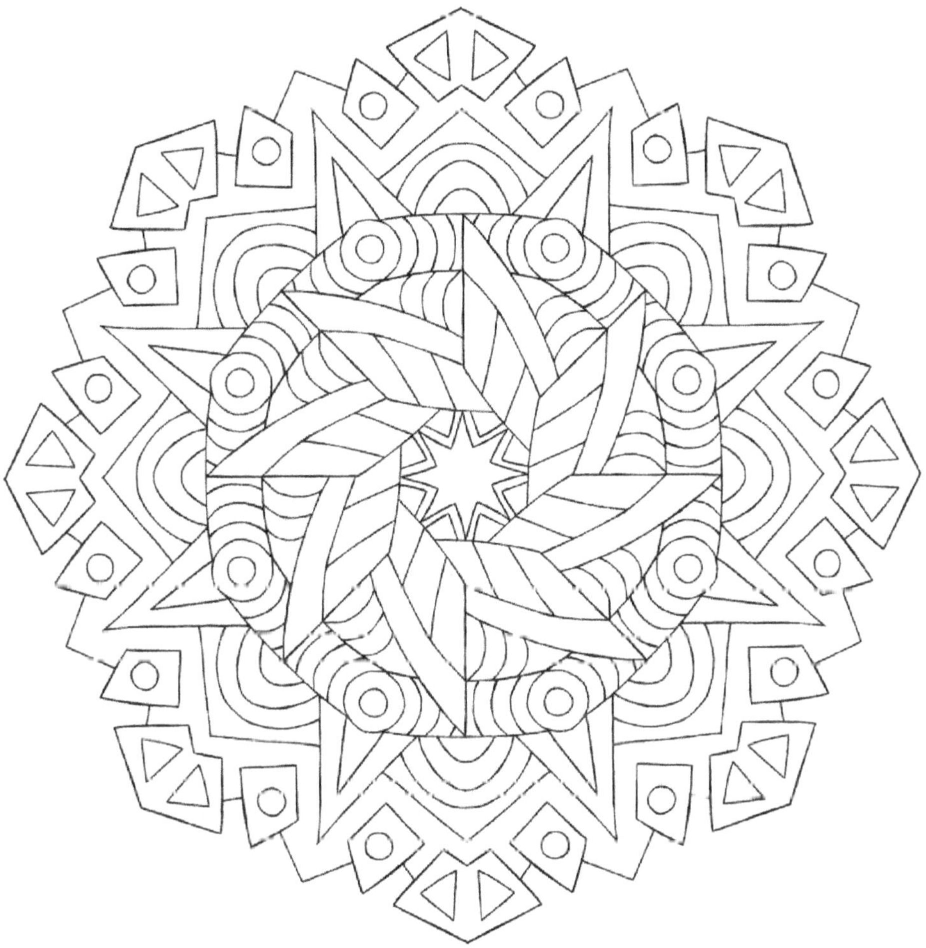

Seek Emotional Support When Needed:

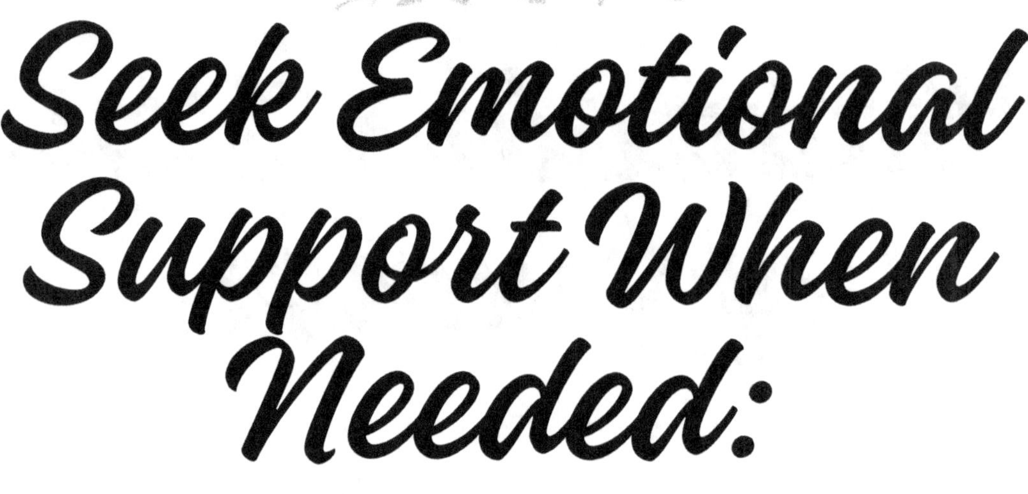

- Don't hesitate to seek professional counseling or therapy if you're facing emotional challenges.
- Sharing your feelings with a mental health professional or a support group can provide valuable insights and coping strategies.

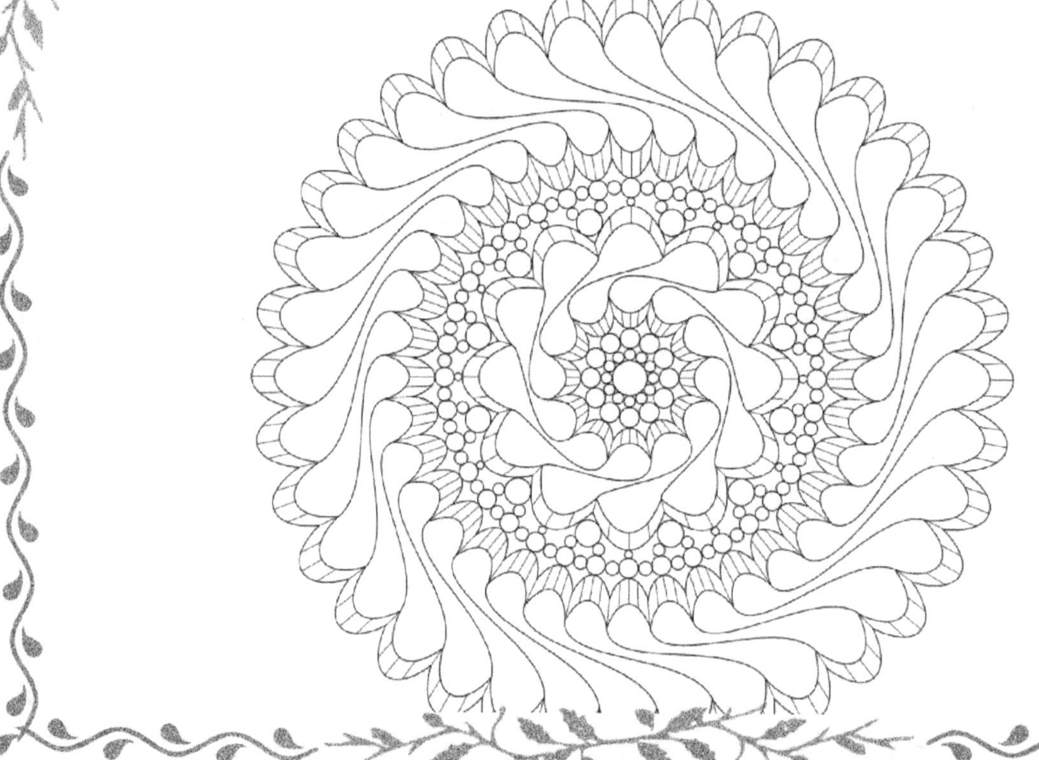

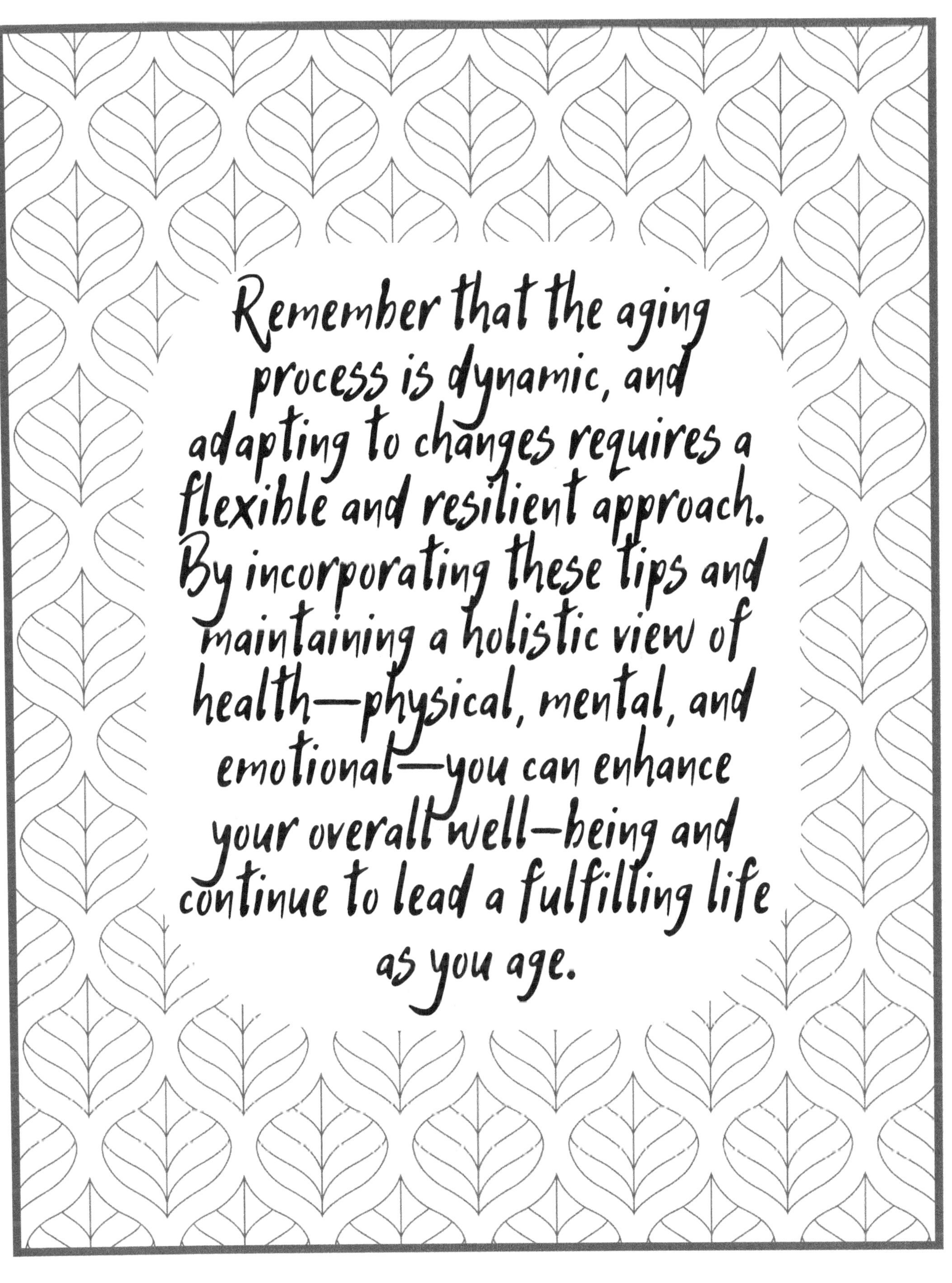

Remember that the aging process is dynamic, and adapting to changes requires a flexible and resilient approach. By incorporating these tips and maintaining a holistic view of health—physical, mental, and emotional—you can enhance your overall well-being and continue to lead a fulfilling life as you age.

Stay Hydrated:

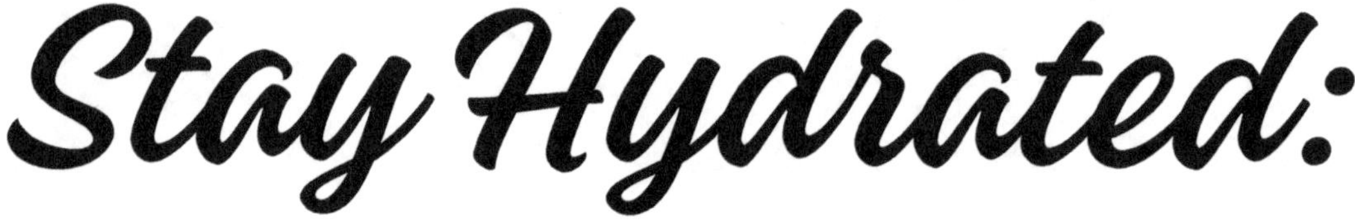

- Adequate hydration is essential for overall health. Drink plenty of water throughout the day to support digestion, circulation, and organ function.
- Limit the intake of dehydrating substances such as caffeine and alcohol.

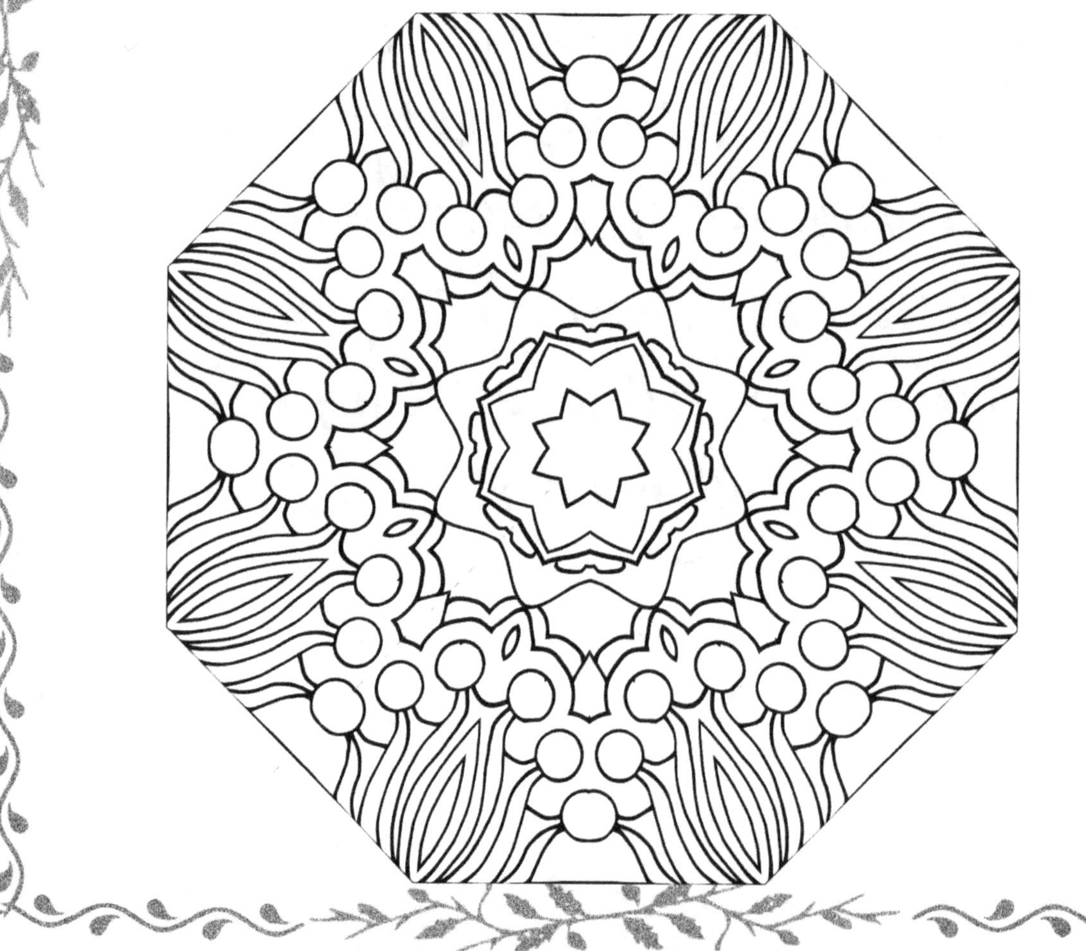

Maintain a Healthy Weight:

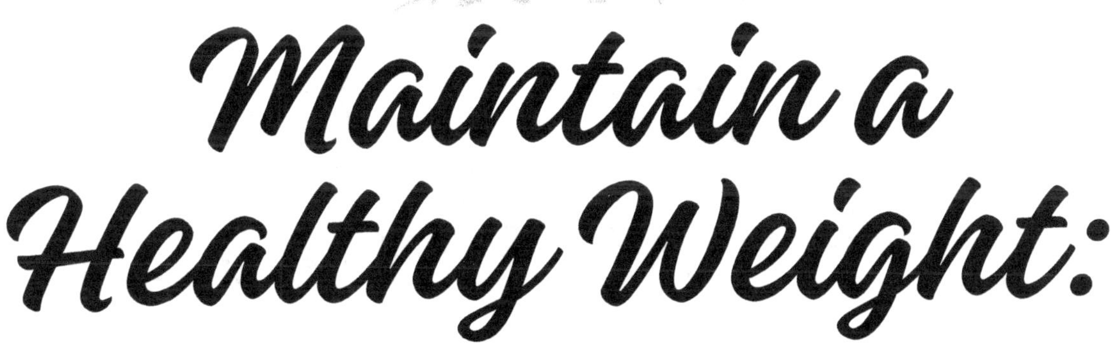

- Strive to maintain a healthy weight to reduce the risk of chronic conditions such as diabetes, heart disease, and joint problems.
- Focus on a well-balanced diet and portion control, and consult with a nutritionist if needed.
-

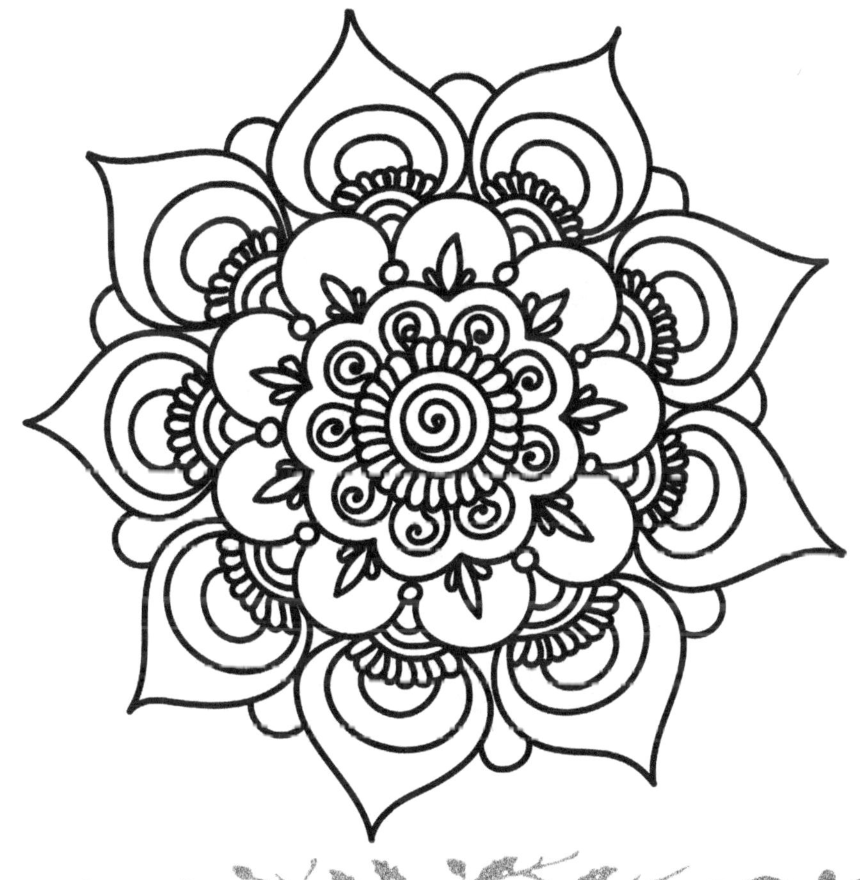

Adapt Your Exercise Routine:

- Modify your exercise routine based on your current physical condition. Low-impact exercises, such as swimming or cycling, can be gentler on joints.
- Incorporate flexibility exercises to improve range of motion and reduce stiffness.

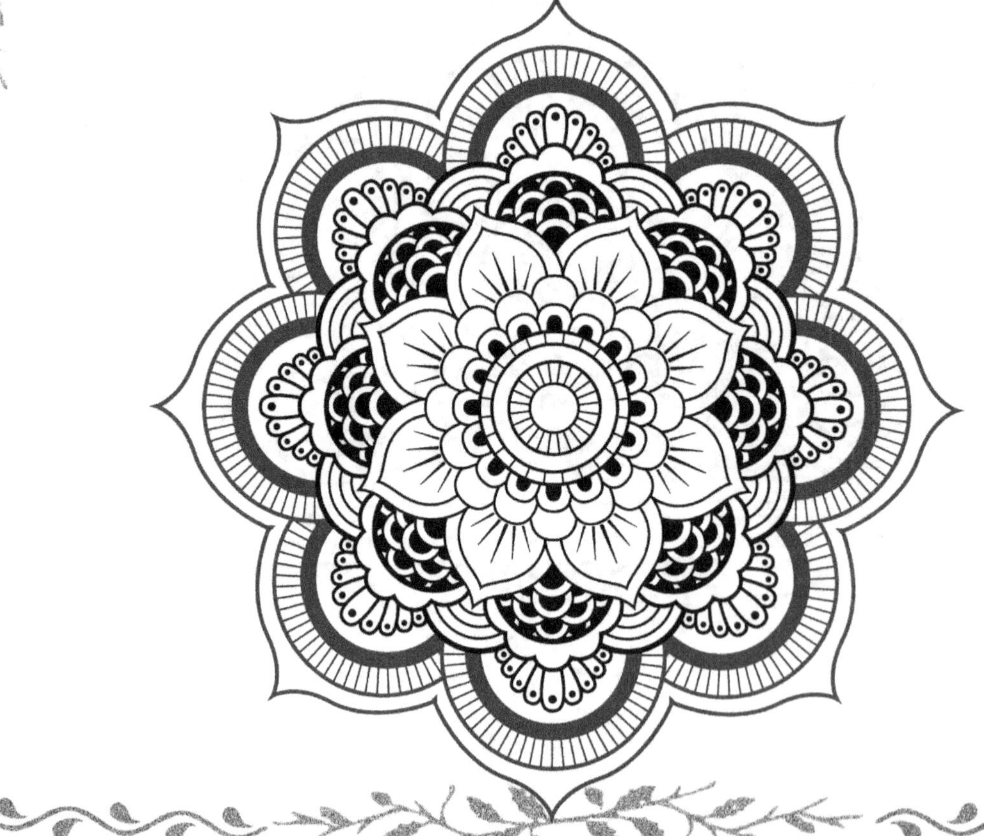

Stay Informed About Medications:

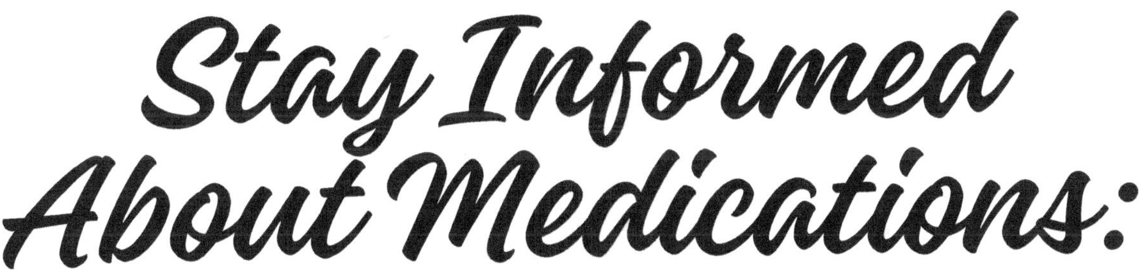

- Be aware of the potential side effects of medications, and communicate with your healthcare provider if you experience any adverse reactions.
- Keep an up-to-date list of medications and share it with all healthcare professionals involved in your care.

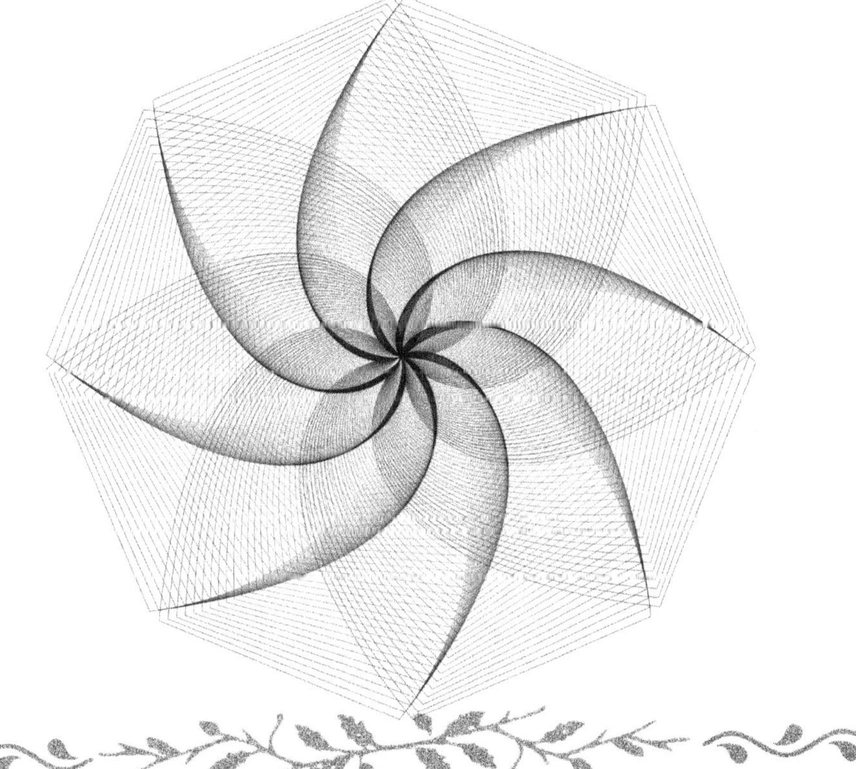

Consider Preventive Measures:

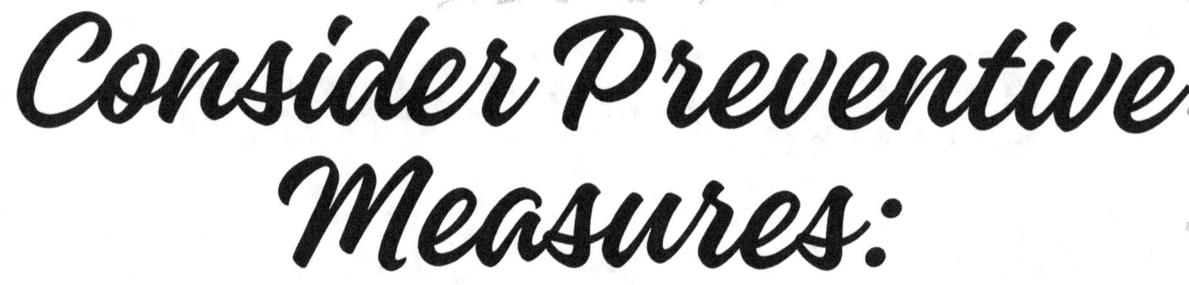

- Stay up-to-date with vaccinations and preventive screenings to catch potential health issues early.
- Practice good hygiene to prevent infections, and follow recommended health guidelines.

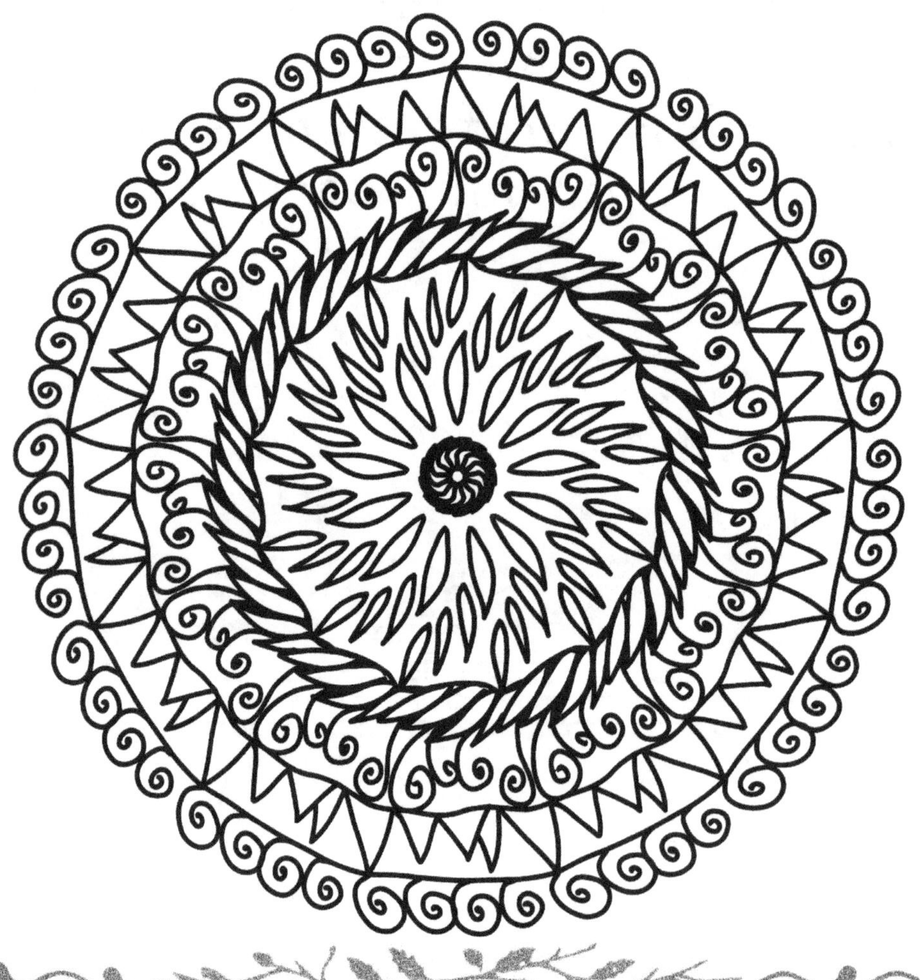

Foster Healthy Relationships:

- Nurture positive relationships with friends, family, and community members.
- Surround yourself with a supportive network that understands your needs and encourages a healthy lifestyle.

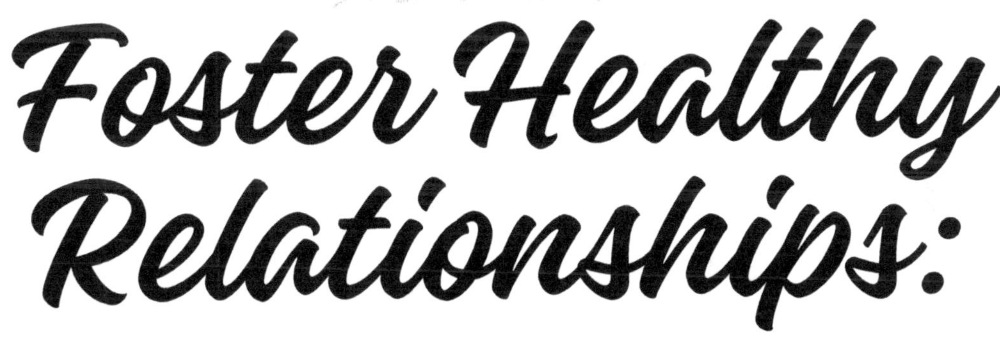

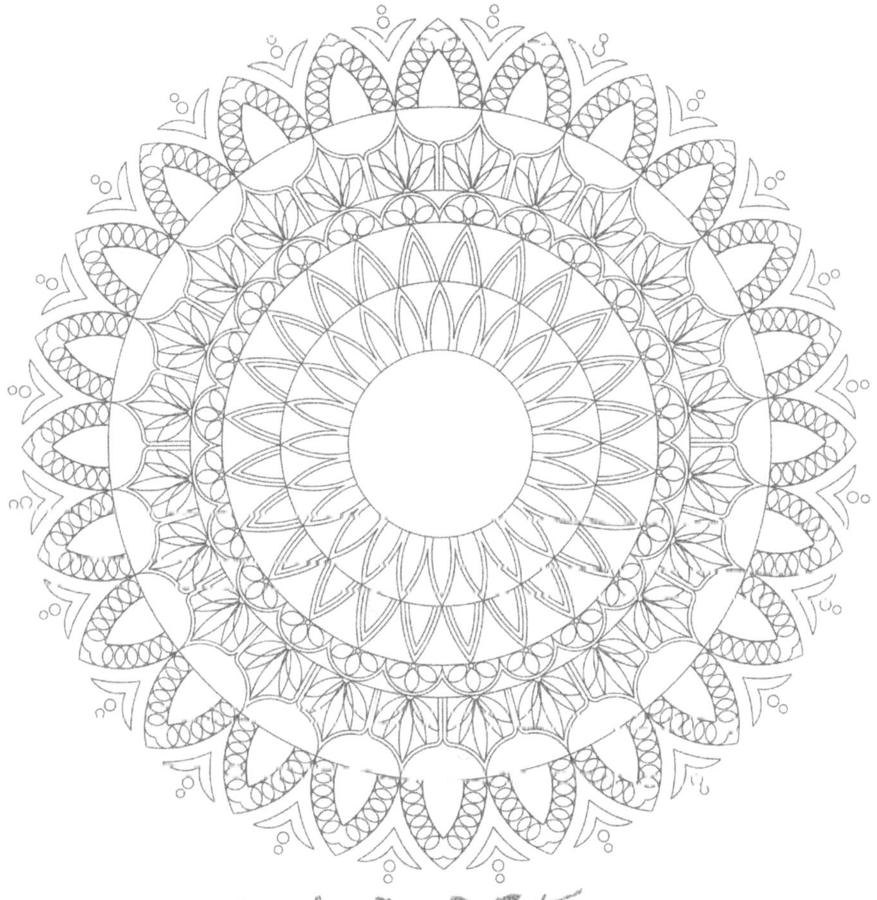

Engage in Creative Outlets:

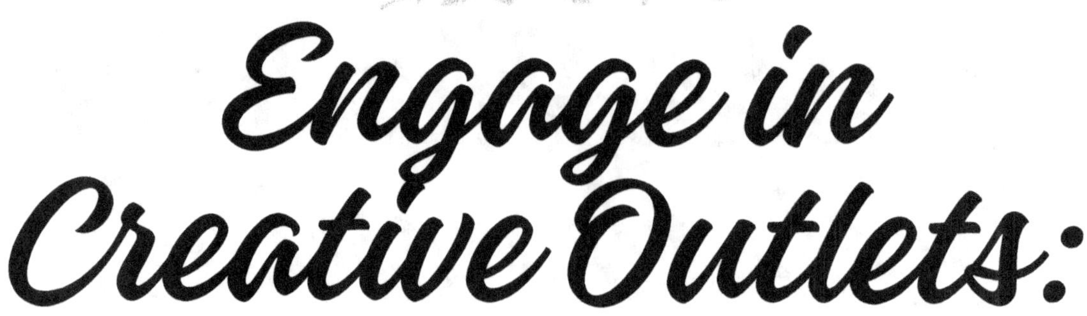

- Explore creative activities such as art, music, or writing to express yourself and stimulate your mind.
- These outlets can provide a sense of accomplishment and contribute to emotional well-being.

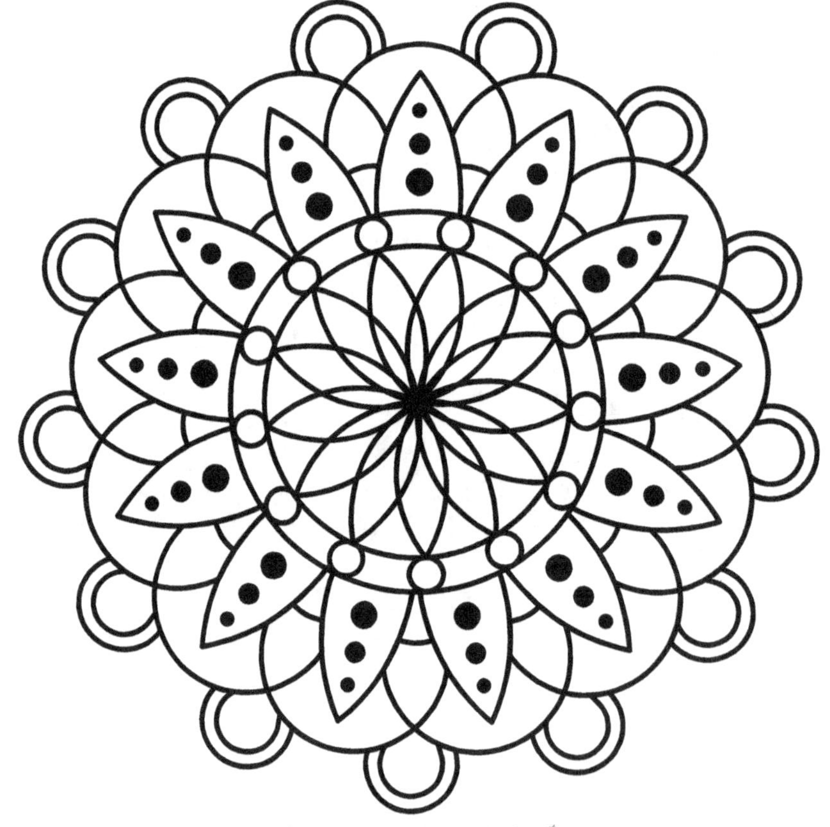

Prioritize Joint Care:

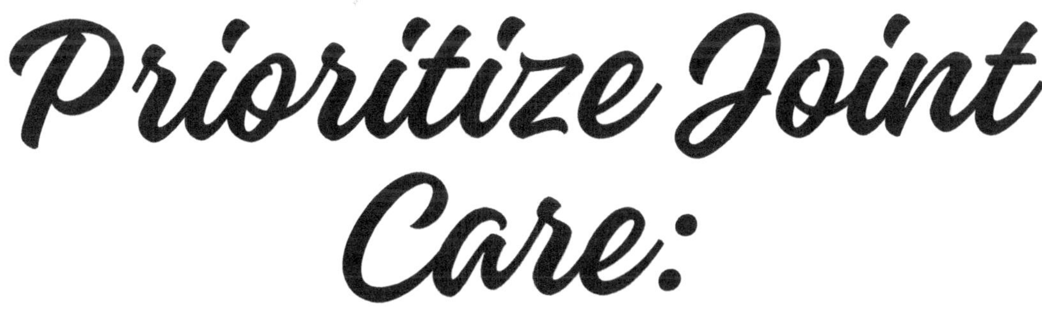

- Be mindful of joint health by avoiding prolonged periods of immobility and maintaining good posture.
- Consider using joint-friendly aids and devices when needed, such as ergonomic chairs or walking aids.

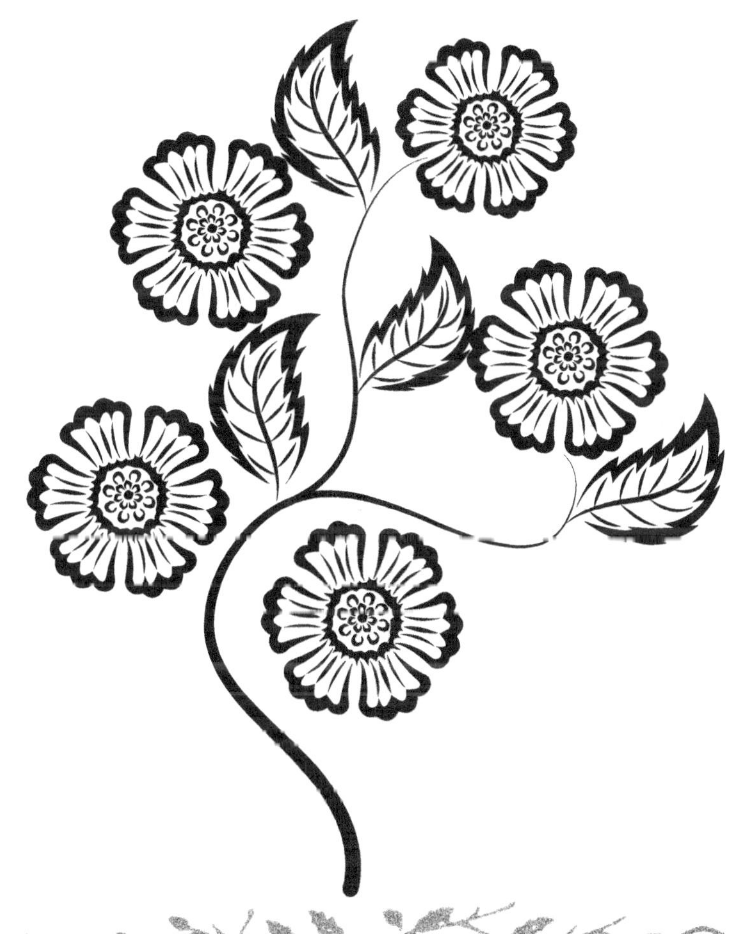

Practice Mindful Eating:

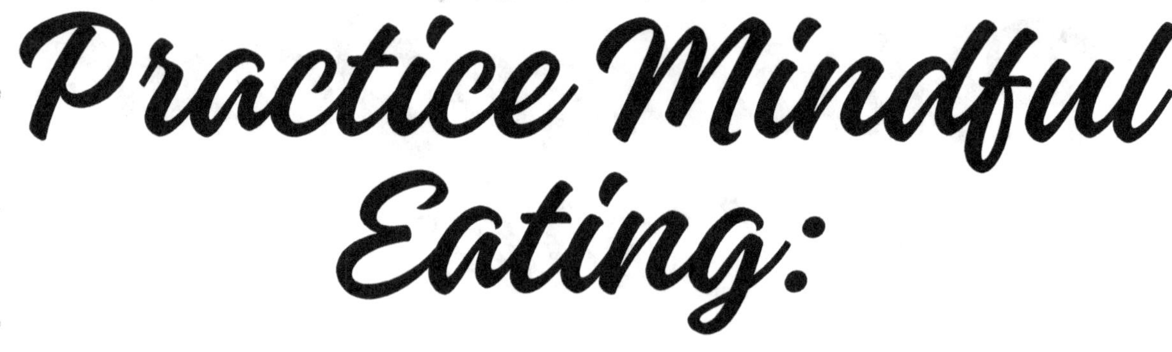

- Pay attention to your eating habits, focusing on mindful eating to savor each bite.
- Listen to your body's hunger and fullness cues, and be conscious of the nutritional value of your meals.

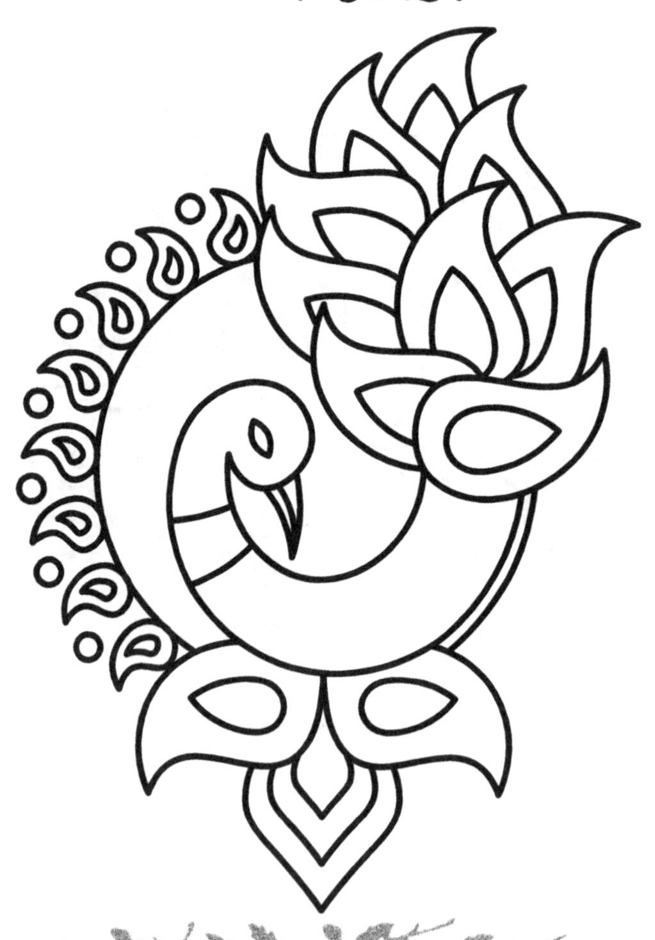

Stay Connected to Nature:

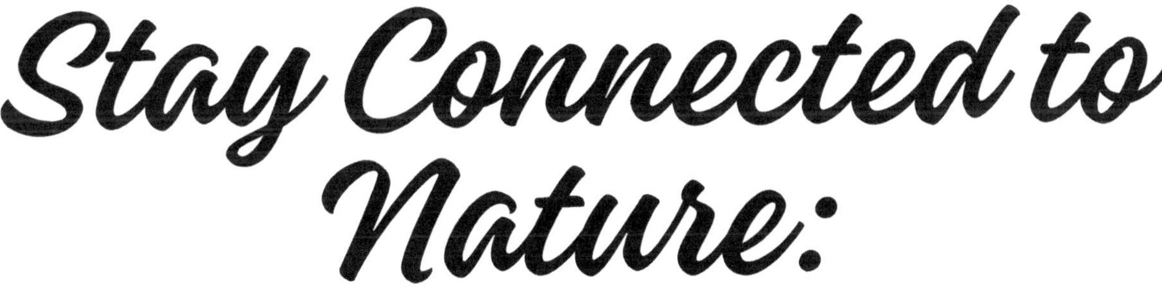

- Spend time outdoors to enjoy the benefits of fresh air, sunlight, and nature.
- Activities such as gardening or leisurely walks in a park can contribute to both physical and mental well-being.

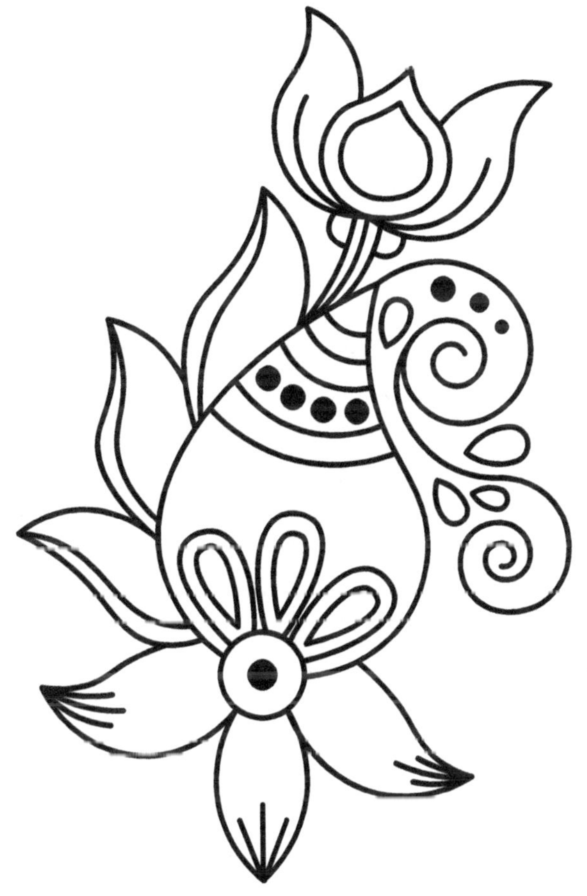

Explore Alternative Therapies:

- Consider alternative therapies such as acupuncture, massage, or herbal remedies to complement traditional medical approaches.
- Consult with healthcare professionals to ensure these therapies align with your health goals.

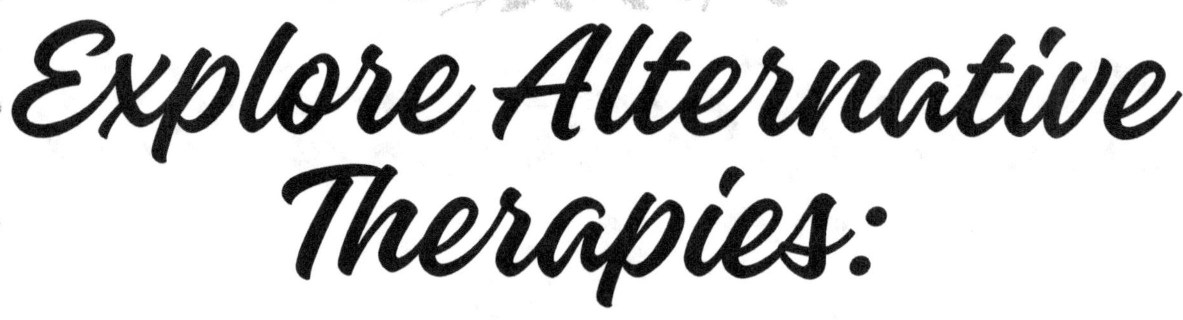

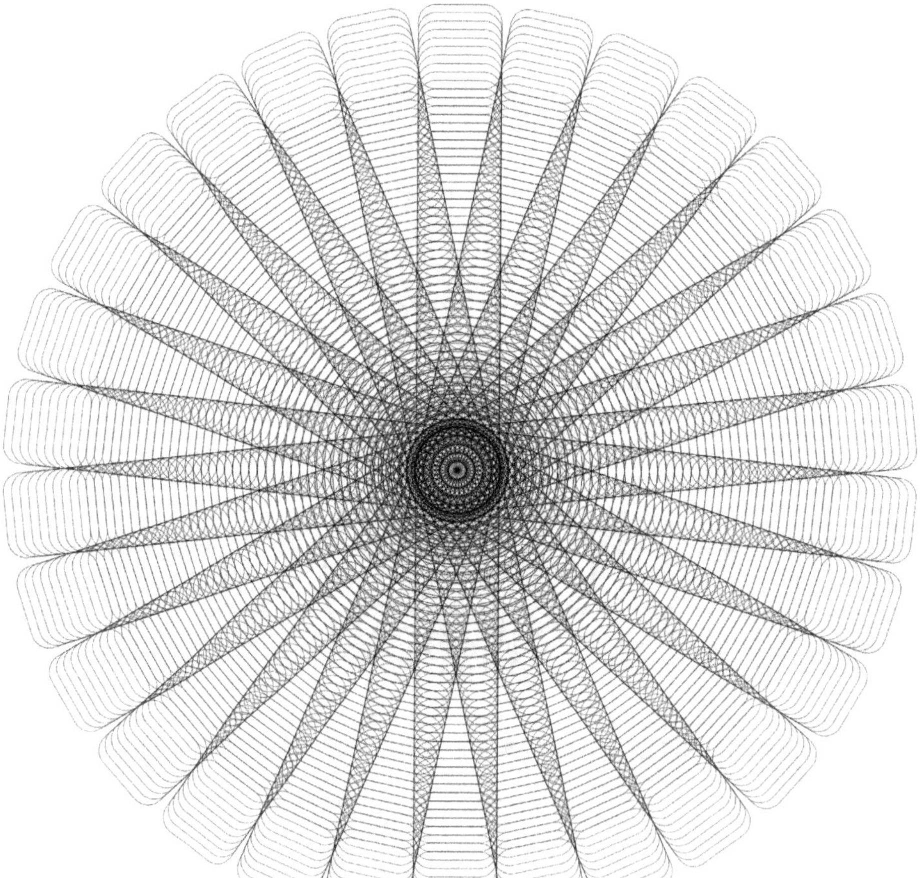

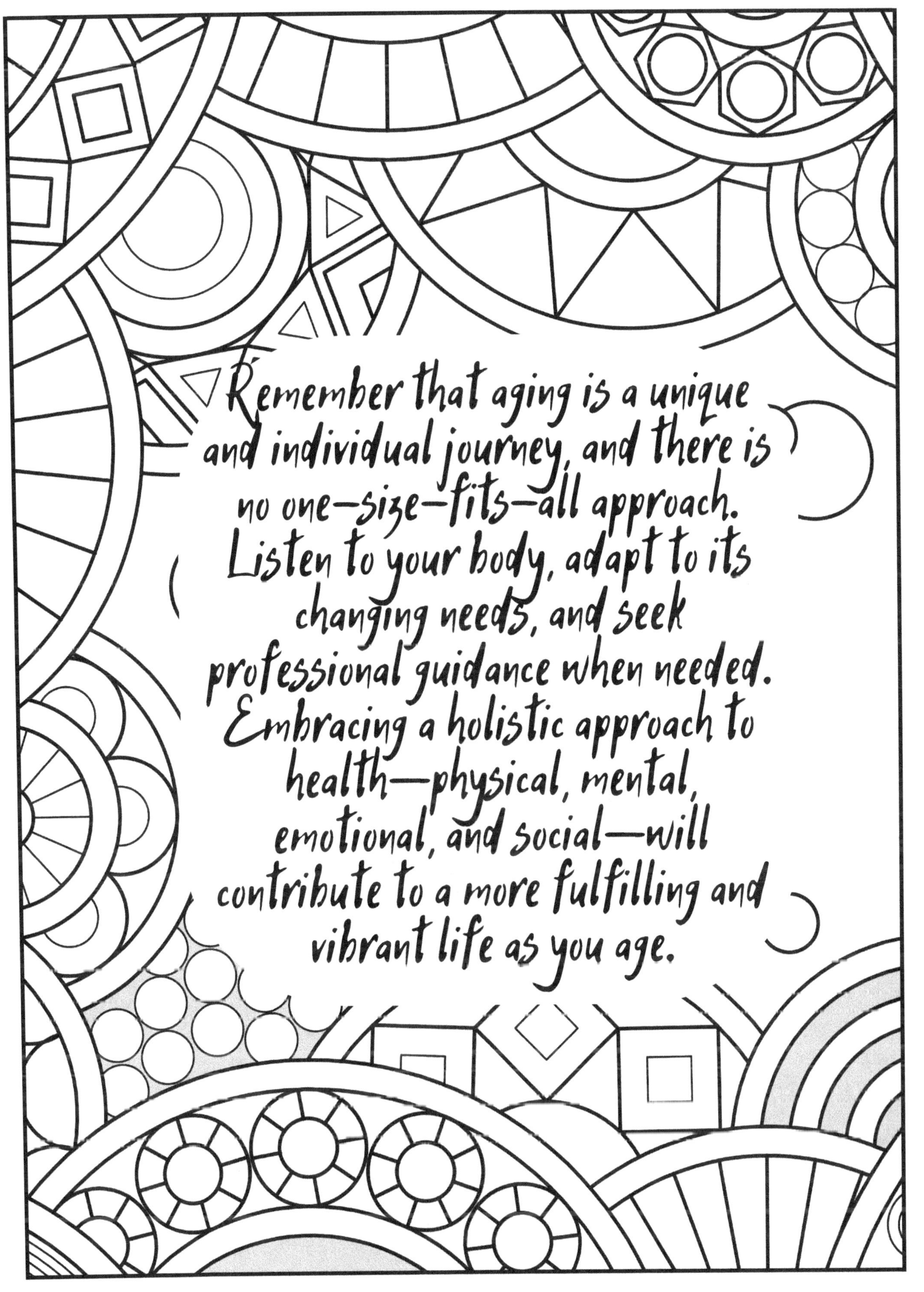

Remember that aging is a unique and individual journey, and there is no one-size-fits-all approach. Listen to your body, adapt to its changing needs, and seek professional guidance when needed. Embracing a holistic approach to health—physical, mental, emotional, and social—will contribute to a more fulfilling and vibrant life as you age.

Embrace Aging Gracefully:

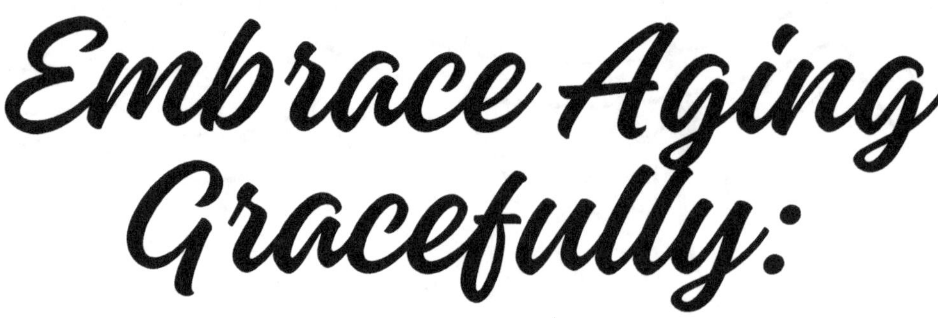

- Accepting the natural aging process with grace can positively impact your mental and emotional well-being.
- Celebrate the wisdom and experiences gained over the years.

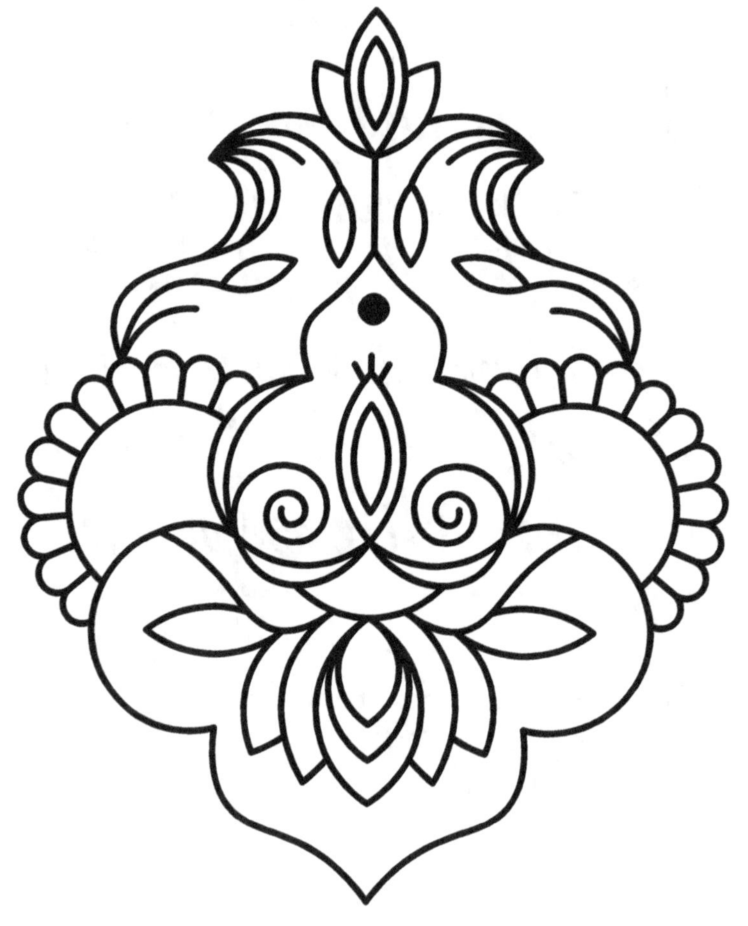

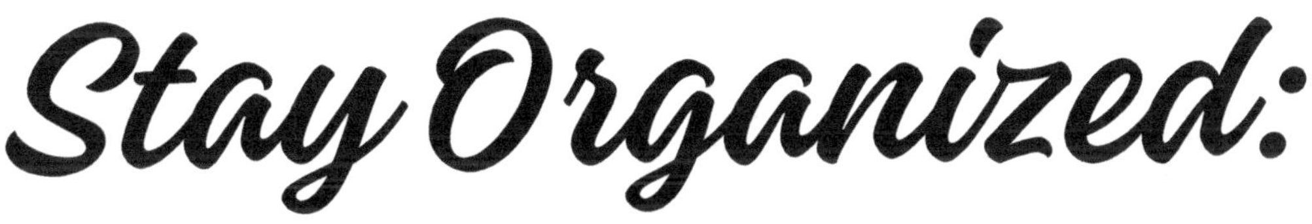

Stay Organized:

- Keep track of appointments, medications, and important health information.
- Use calendars, planners, or smartphone apps to stay organized and ensure you are managing your health effectively.

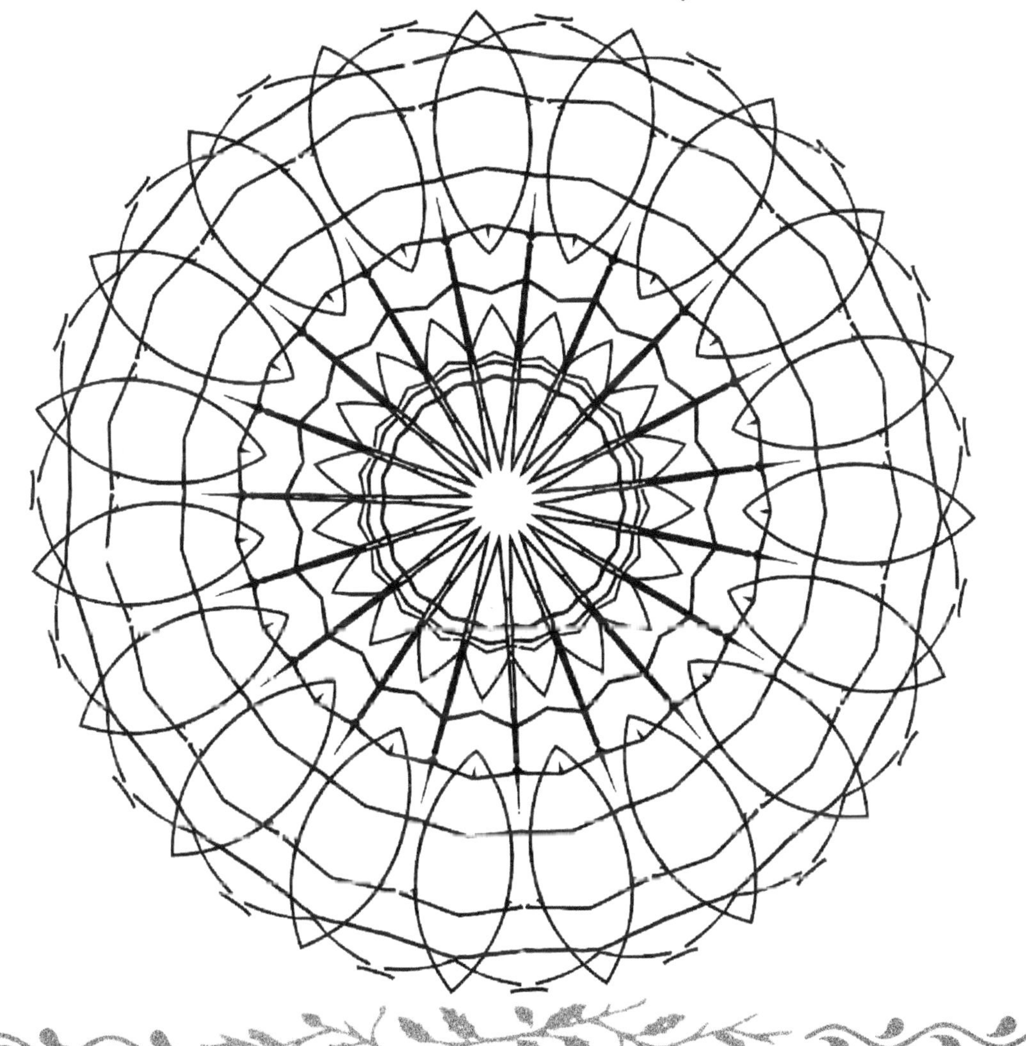

Cognitive Exercises:

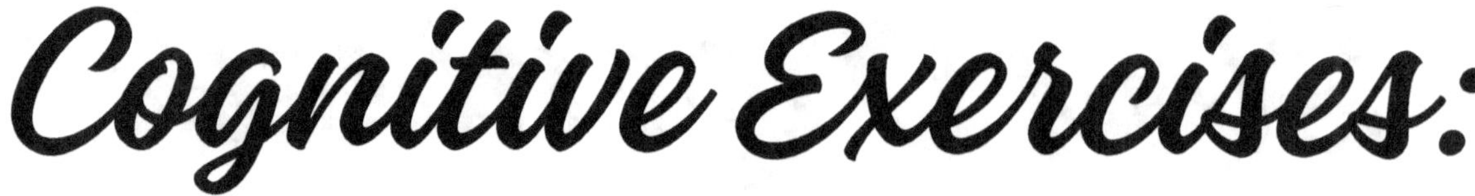

- Engage in activities that challenge your cognitive abilities, such as puzzles, memory games, and learning new skills.
- Continued mental stimulation can help support cognitive function and maintain a sharp mind.

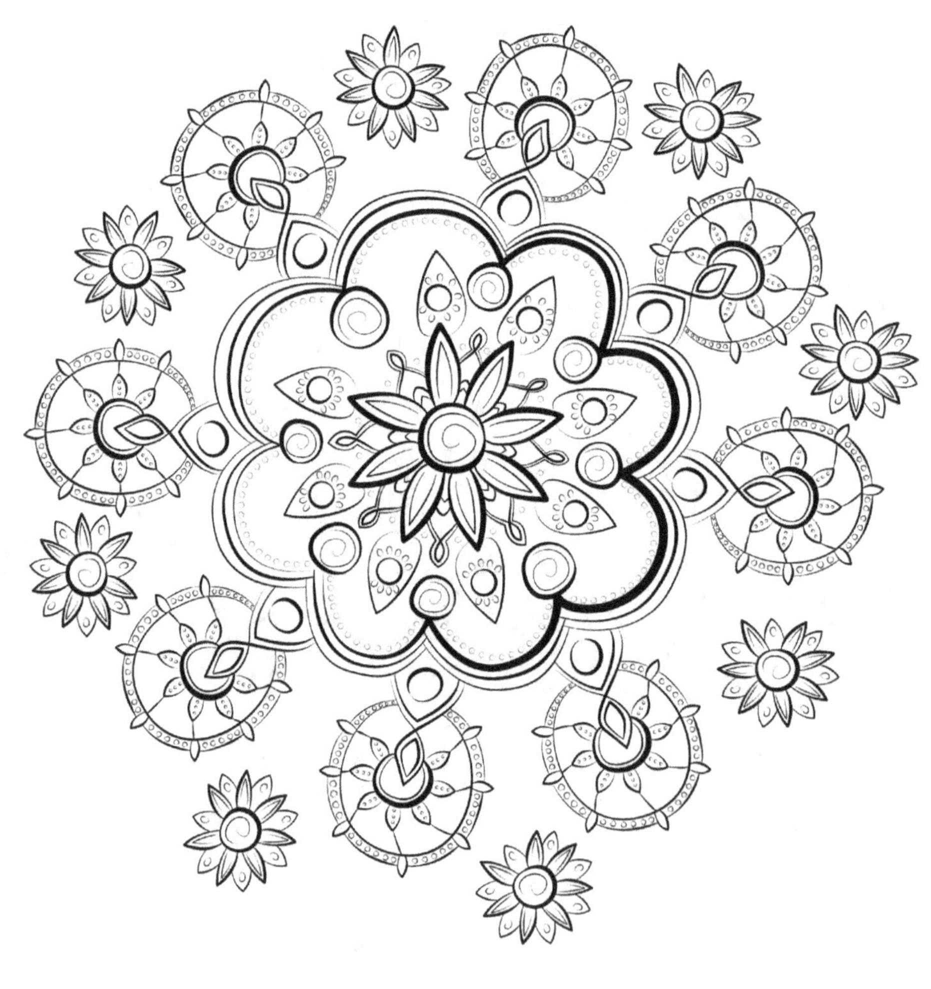

Stay Involved in Community Activities:

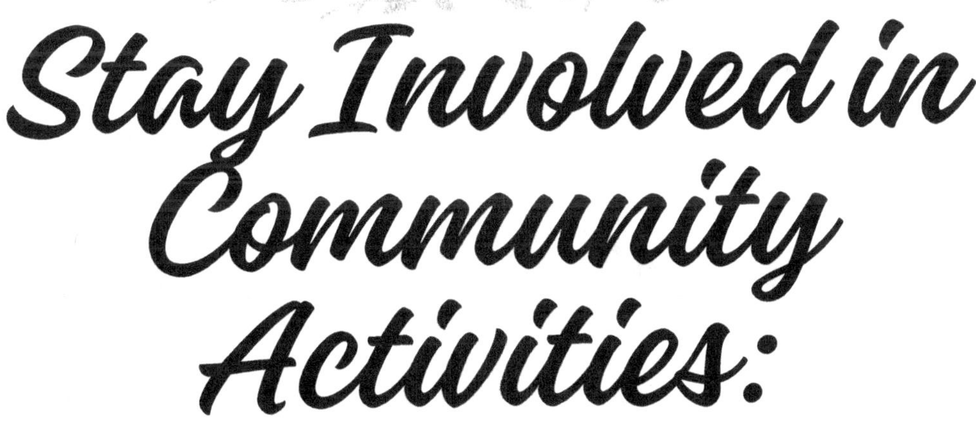

- Participate in community events, social groups, or clubs that align with your interests.
- Engaging in community activities provides opportunities for social interaction and a sense of belonging.

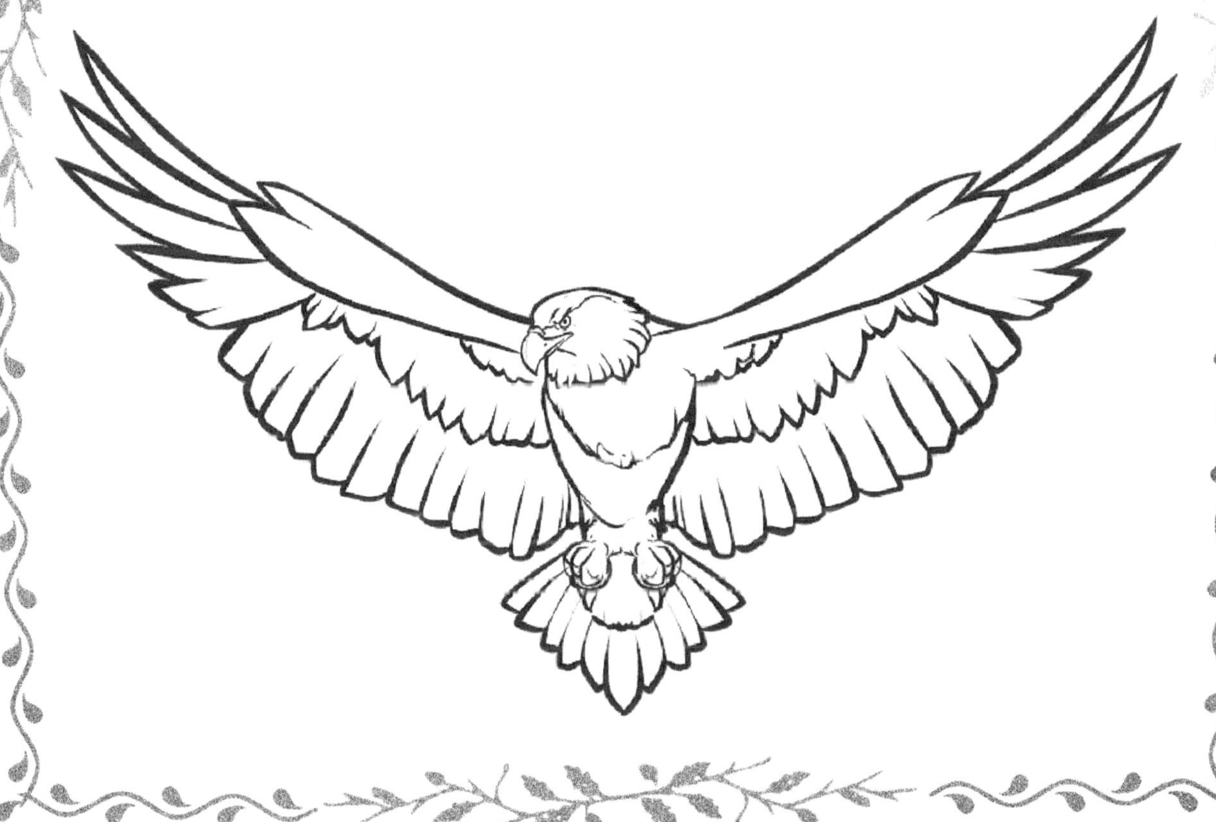

Maintain a Healthy Mouth:

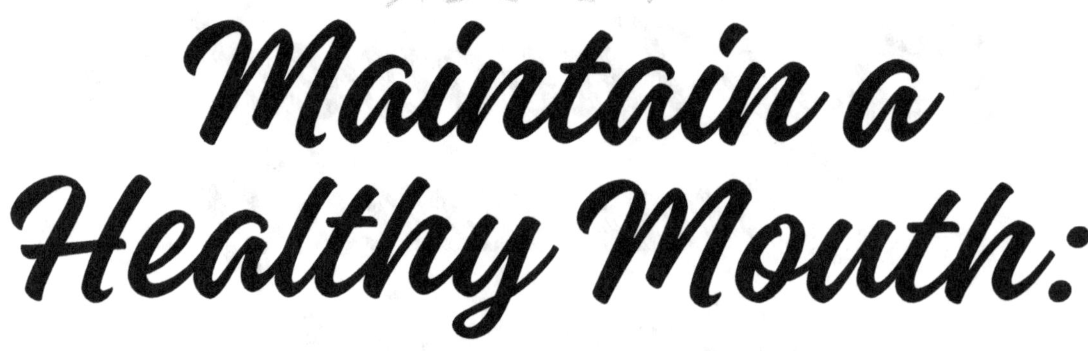

- Oral health is crucial for overall well-being. Brush and floss regularly, and schedule regular dental check-ups.
- Address dental issues promptly to prevent complications that can impact your overall health.

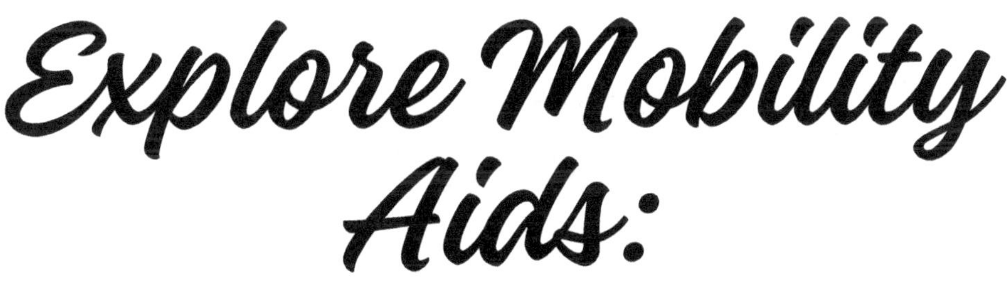

Explore Mobility Aids:

- If mobility becomes a challenge, consider using aids such as canes, walkers, or wheelchairs.
- These tools can enhance independence and safety, allowing you to maintain an active lifestyle.

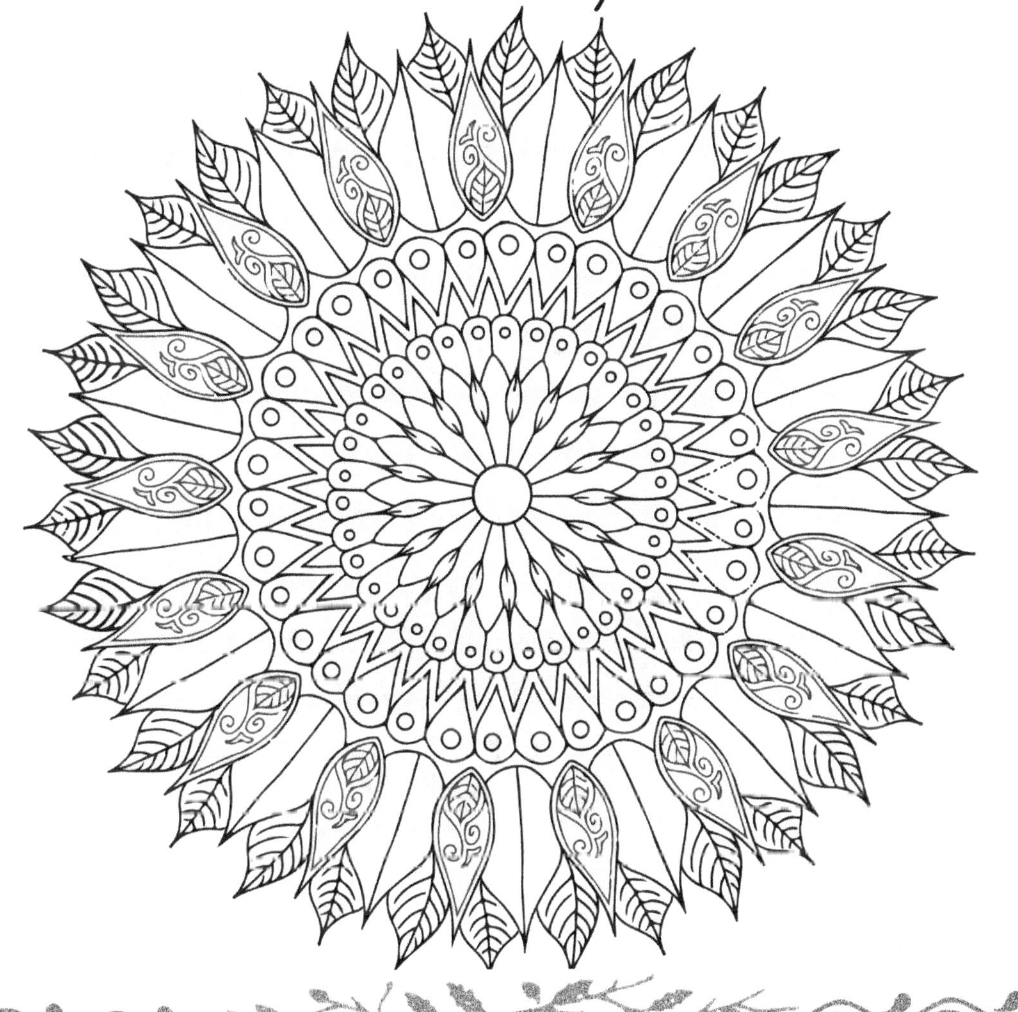

Adopt Stress-Reducing Techniques:

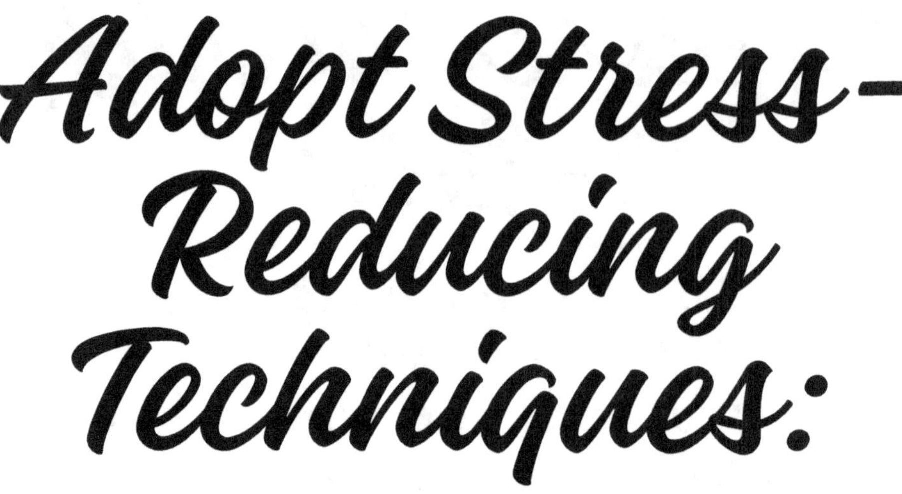

- Practice stress-reducing techniques such as meditation, deep breathing exercises, or progressive muscle relaxation.
- Managing stress is essential for overall health and can positively impact physical and mental well-being..

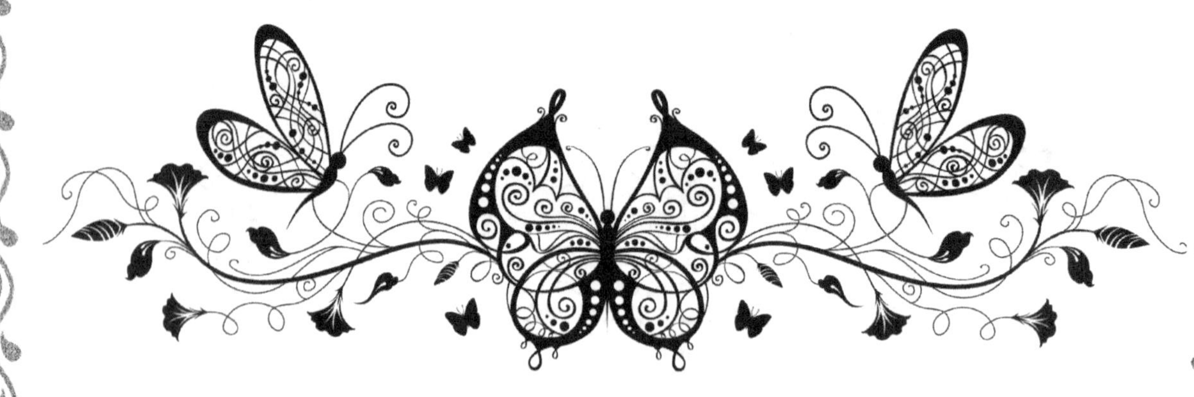

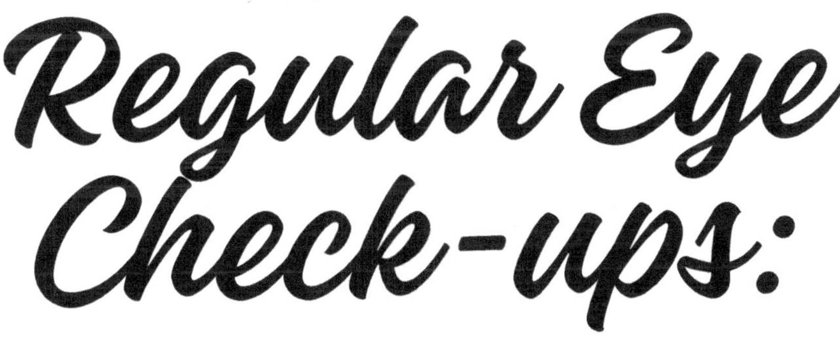

Regular Eye Check-ups:

- Schedule regular eye exams to monitor vision changes and address any issues promptly.
- Good vision is crucial for safety and independence, especially as you navigate your daily activities.

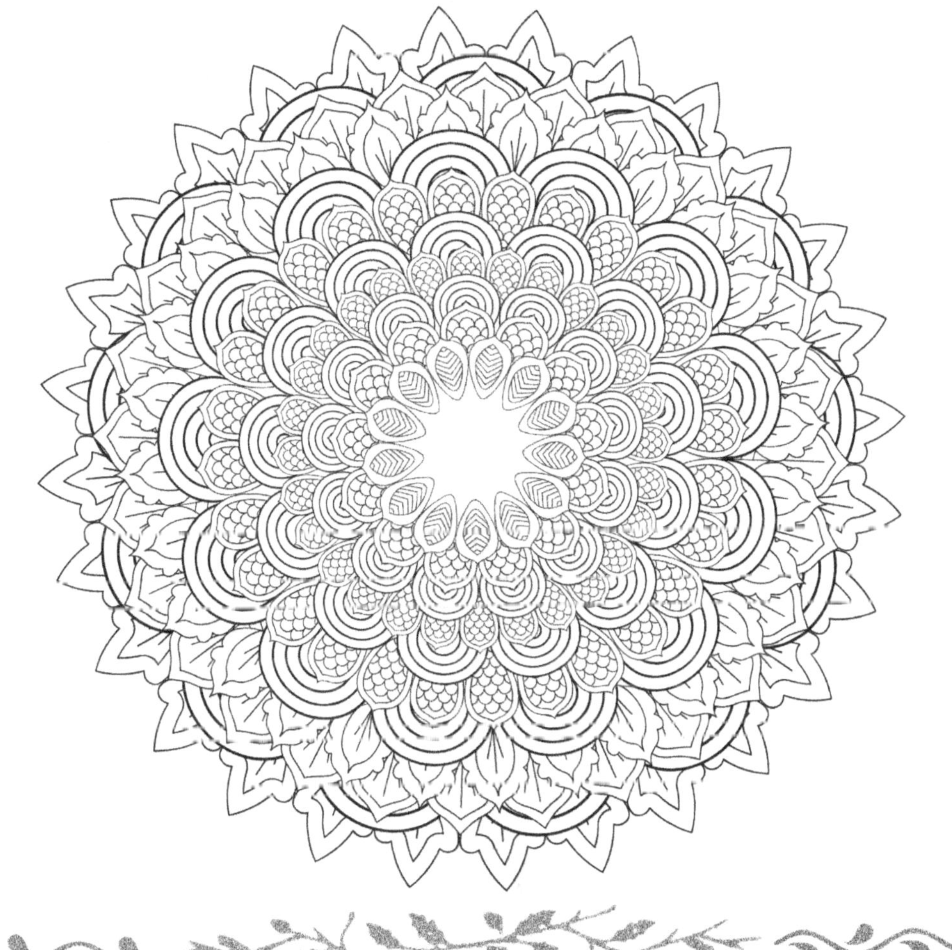

Celebrate Milestones and Memories:

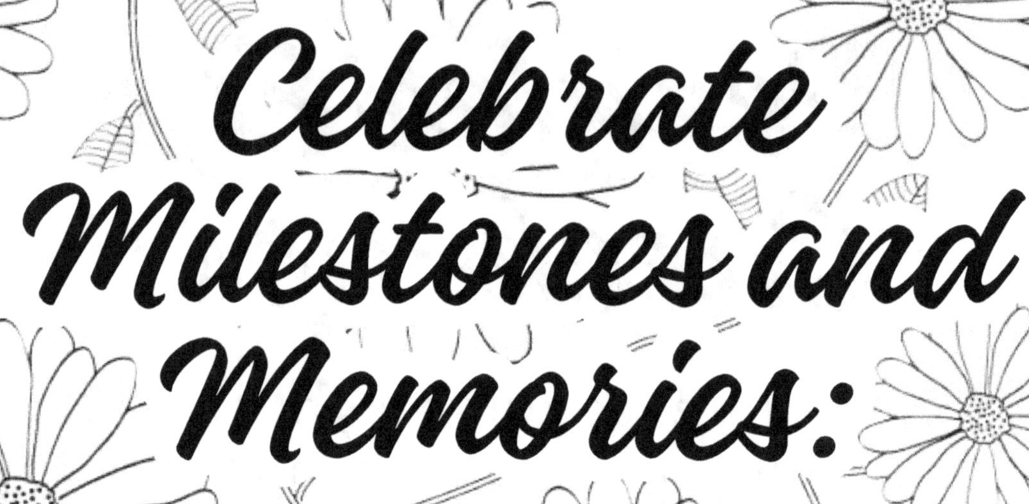

- Take time to reflect on and celebrate significant milestones and memories in your life.
- This reflection can bring a sense of accomplishment and gratitude.

Adapt Your Living Space:

- Make necessary modifications to your home to ensure it is safe and accessible.
- Install handrails, ramps, or other aids to accommodate changing physical needs.

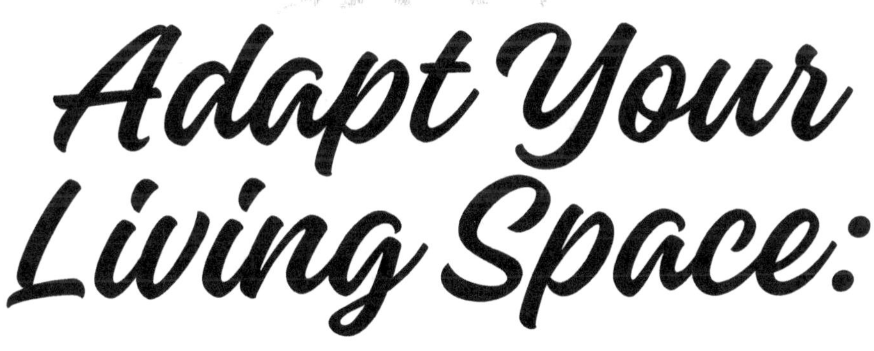

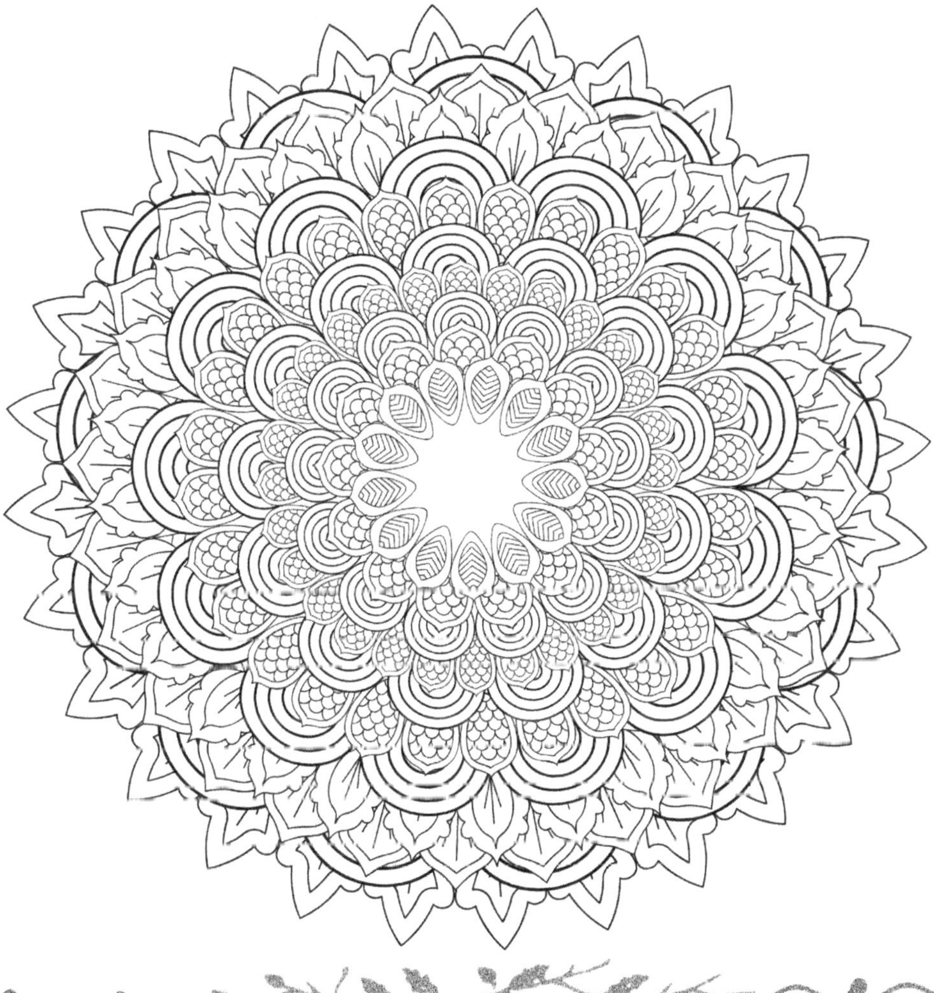

Practice Gratitude:

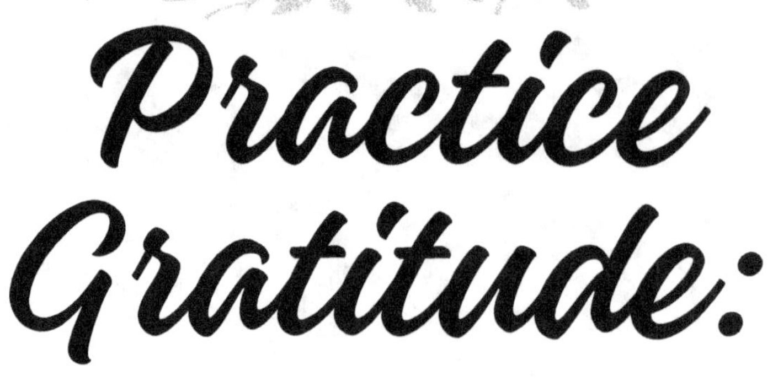

- Cultivate a practice of gratitude by acknowledging and appreciating the positive aspects of your life.
- Focusing on gratitude can contribute to a positive outlook and mental well-being.

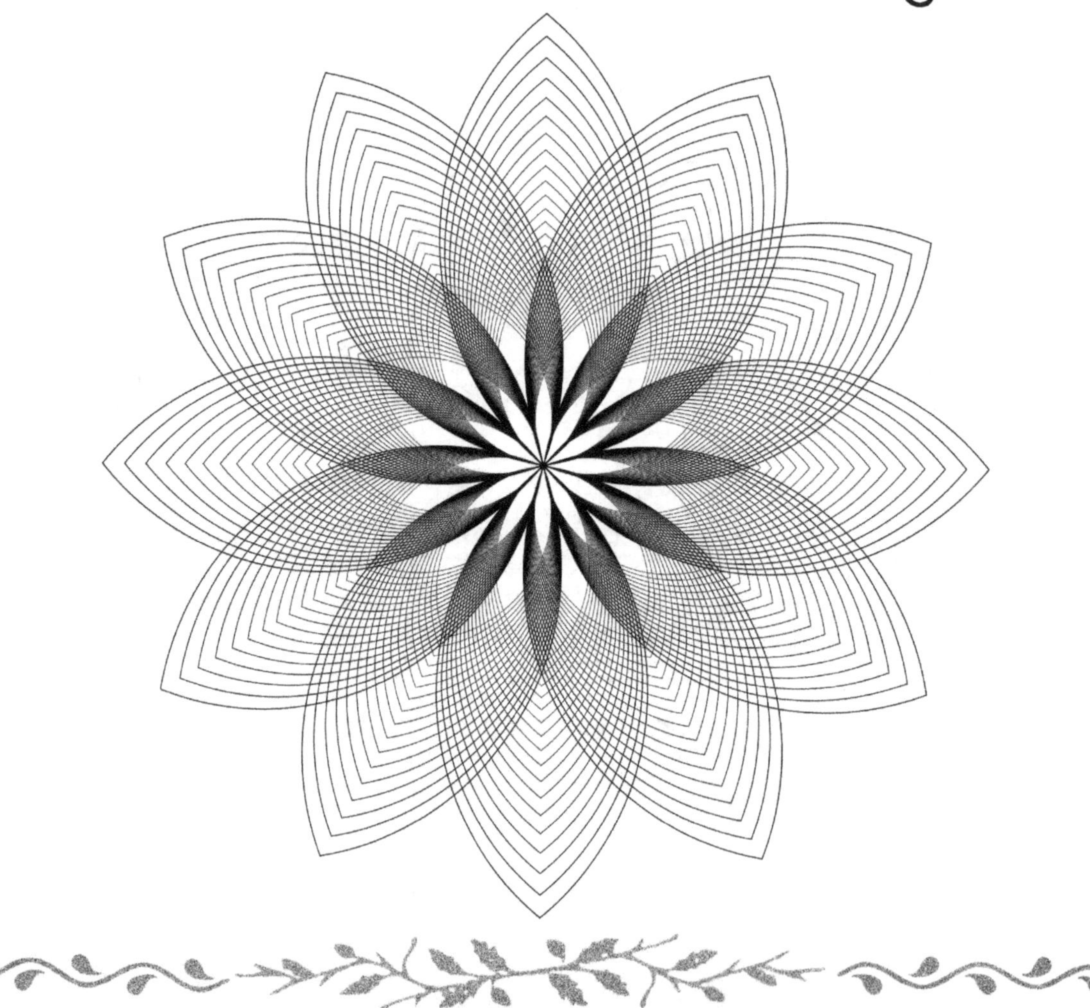

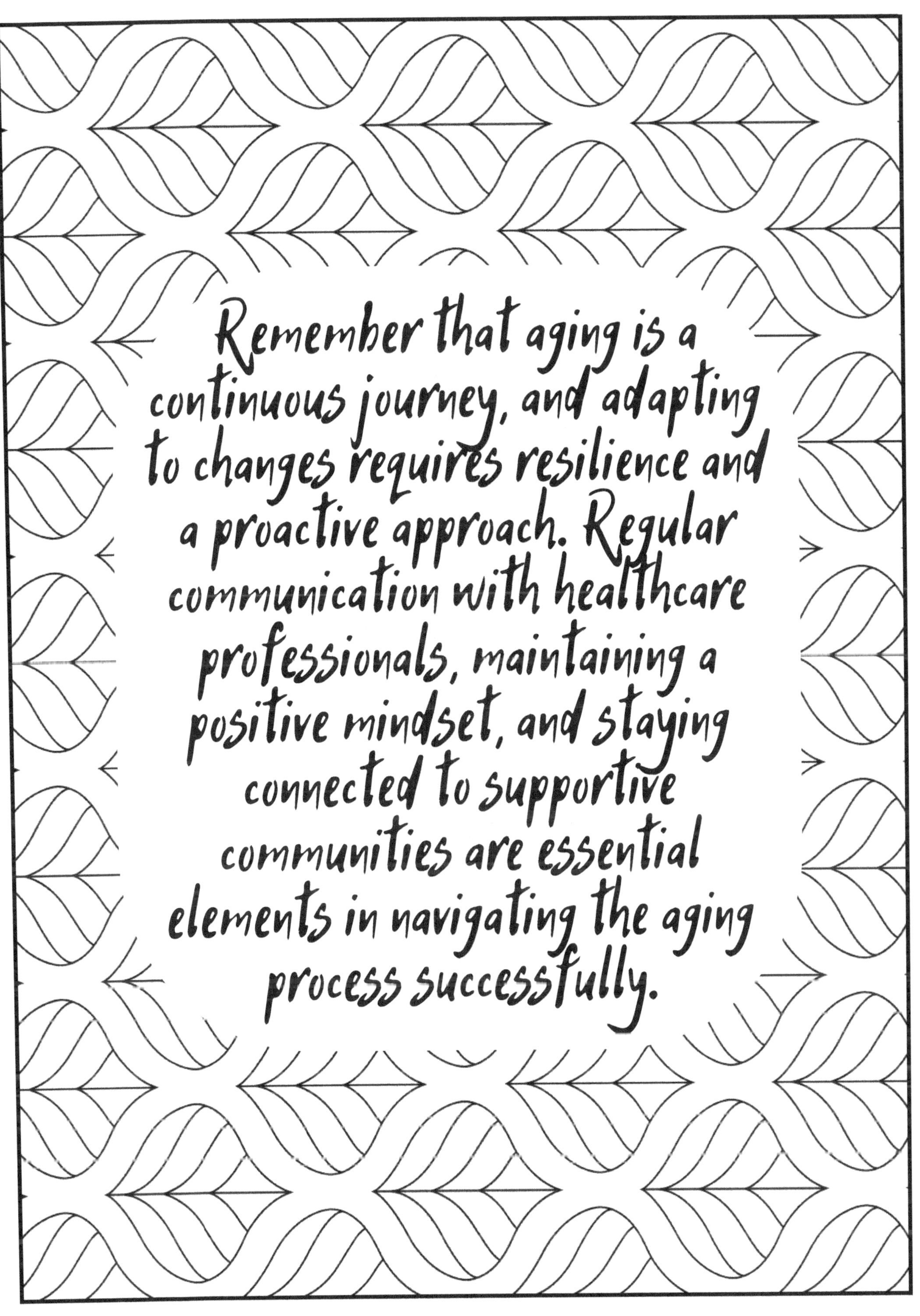

Remember that aging is a continuous journey, and adapting to changes requires resilience and a proactive approach. Regular communication with healthcare professionals, maintaining a positive mindset, and staying connected to supportive communities are essential elements in navigating the aging process successfully.

Stay Informed About Mental Health:

- Be aware of the signs of mental health issues and seek professional help if needed.
- Mental health is an integral part of overall well-being, and early intervention can be crucial.

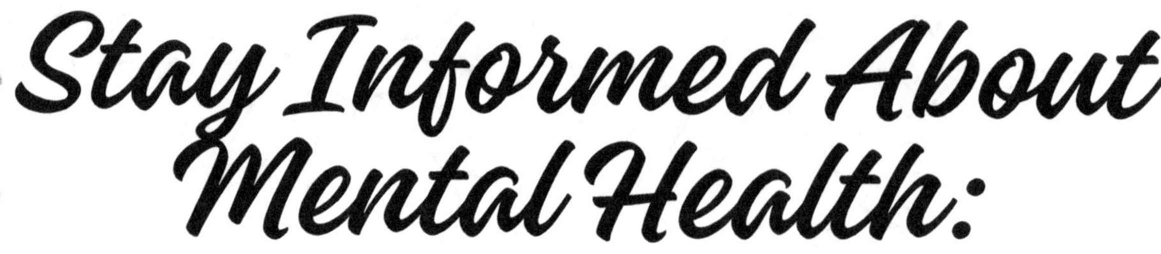

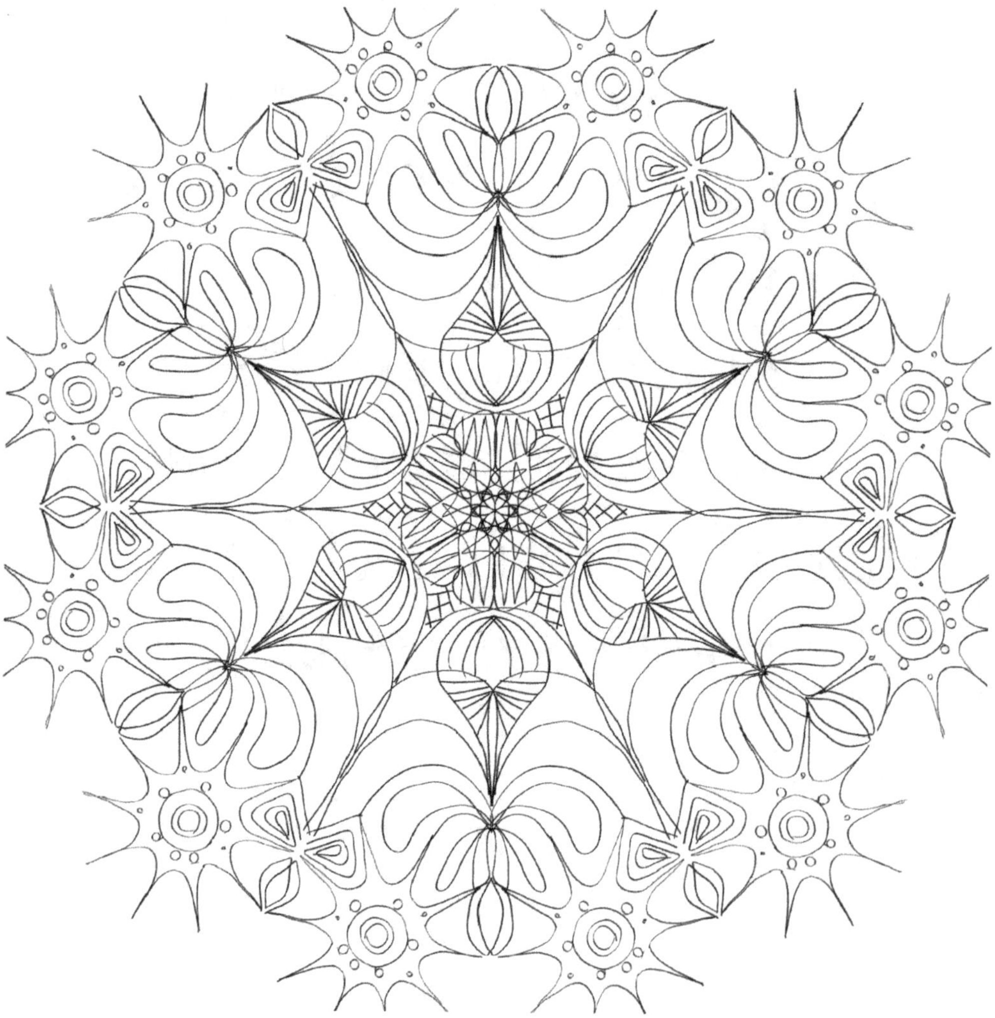

Explore Holistic Therapies:

- Consider holistic therapies such as acupuncture, aromatherapy, or yoga to promote overall wellness.
- These approaches can address physical, mental, and emotional aspects of health.

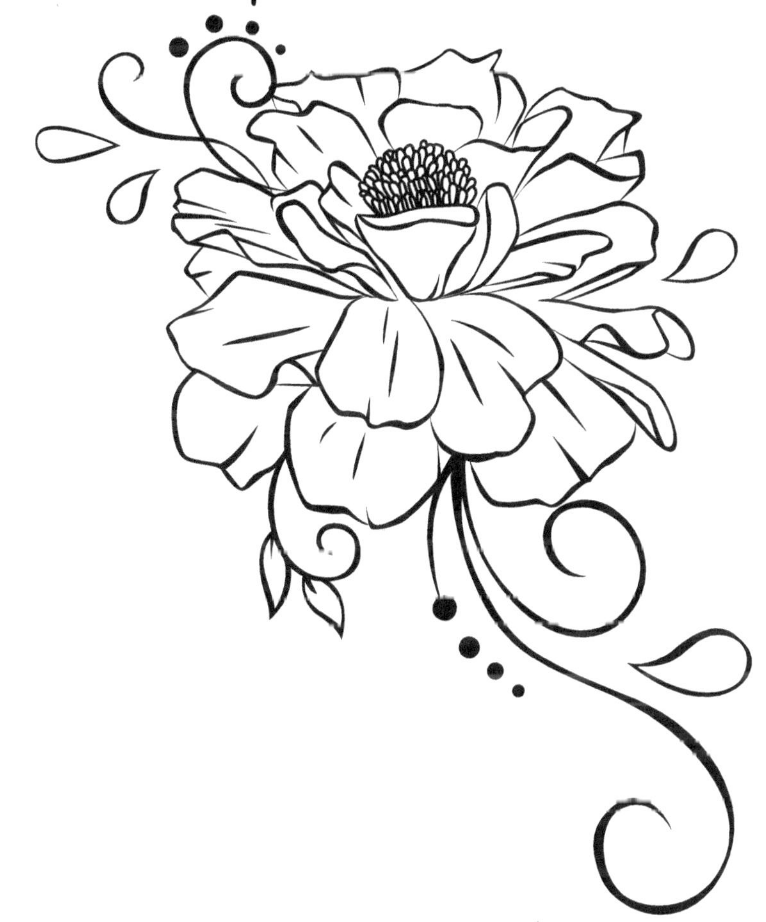

Maintain a Sense of Independence:

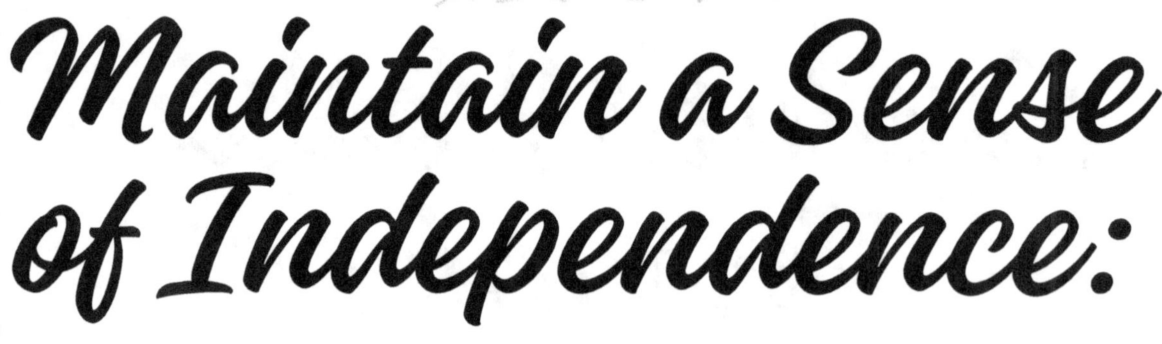

- Strive to maintain a sense of independence in your daily activities.
- Seek assistance when needed, but also focus on tasks that you can still manage on your own.

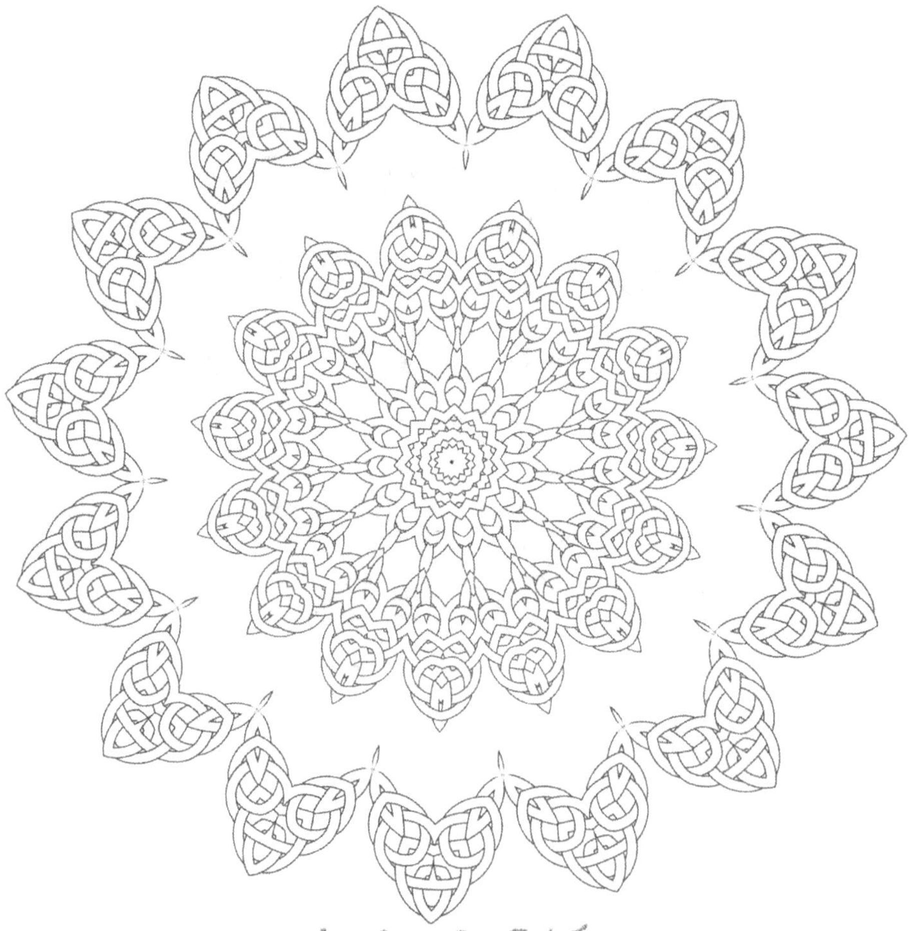

Stay Tech-Savvy:

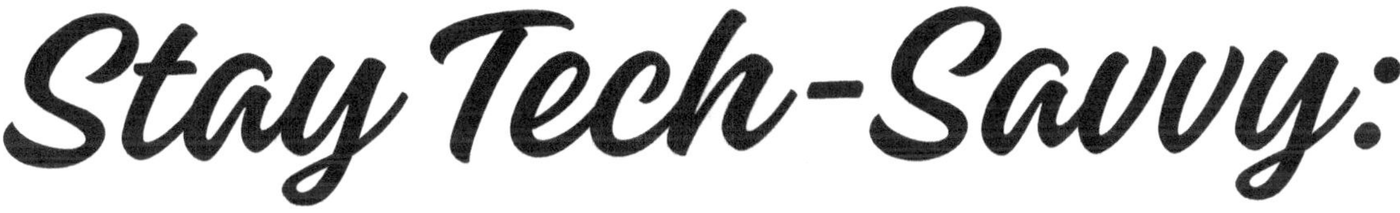

- Embrace technology to stay connected with loved ones, access health information, and engage in online activities.
- Learn to use devices that can enhance your daily life, such as smartphones, tablets, or wearable health trackers.

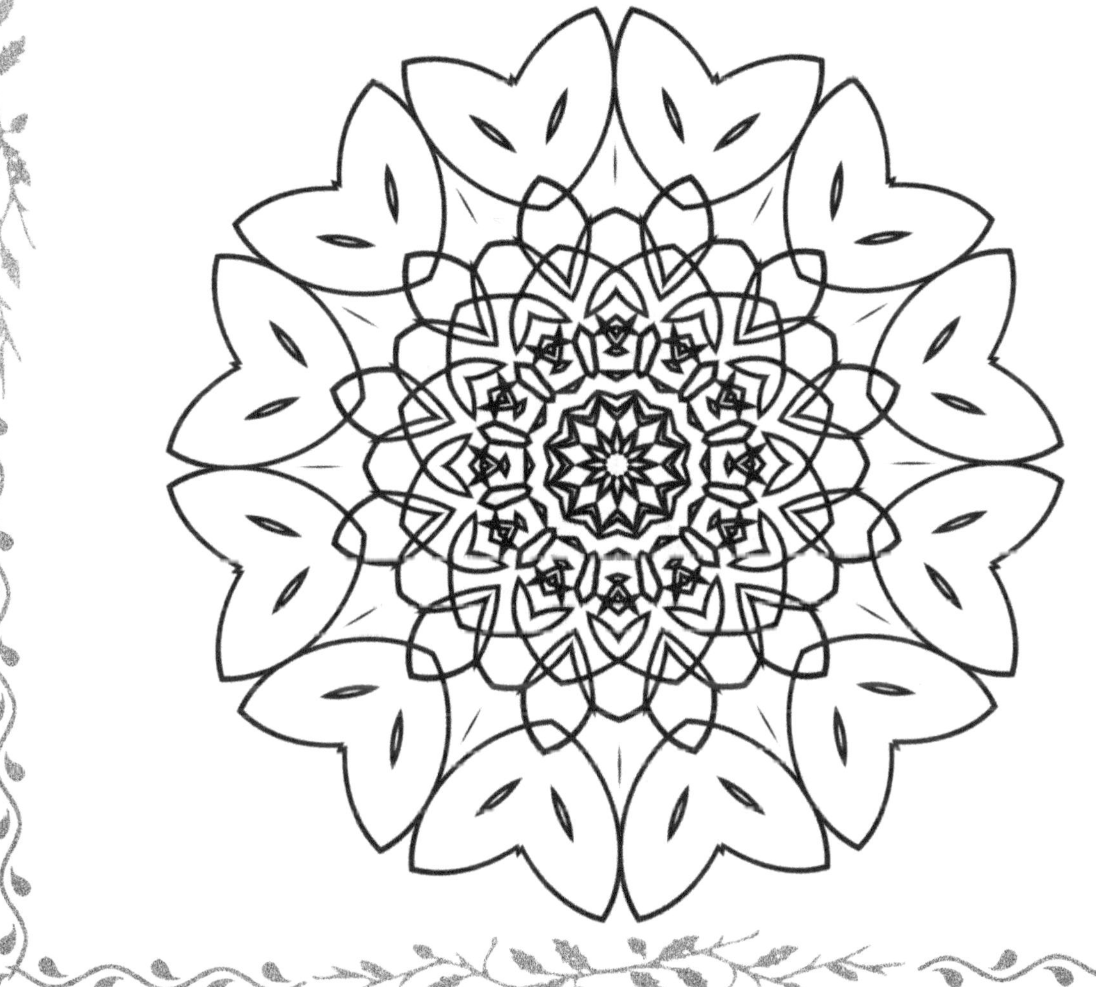

Maintain a Healthy Heart:

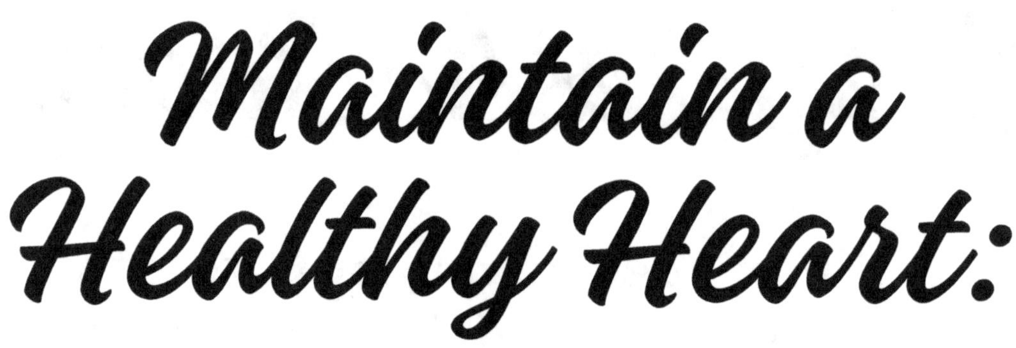

- Prioritize cardiovascular health by incorporating heart-friendly foods into your diet, such as fruits, vegetables, and lean proteins.
- Engage in aerobic exercises like walking, cycling, or swimming to support heart health.

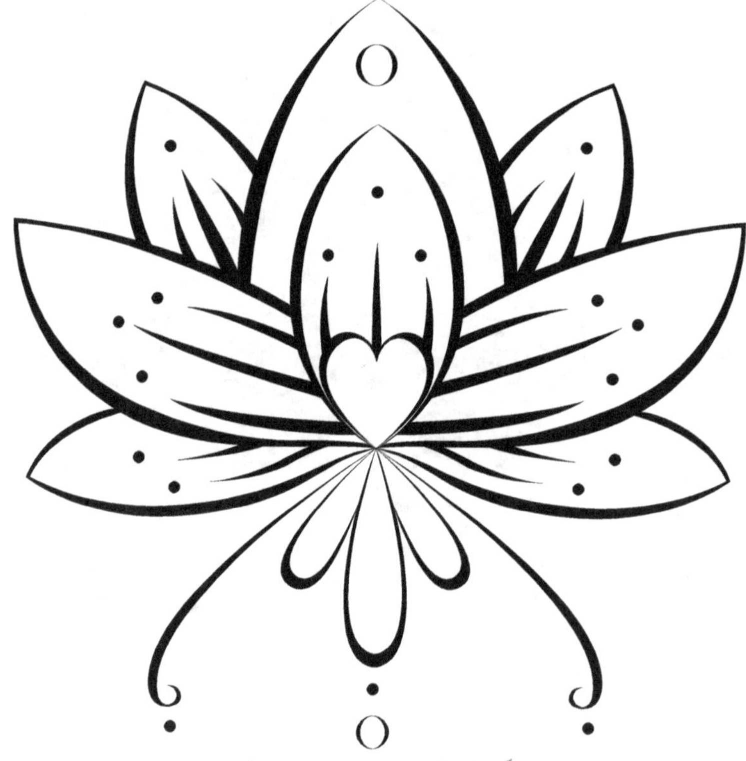

Stay Vaccinated:

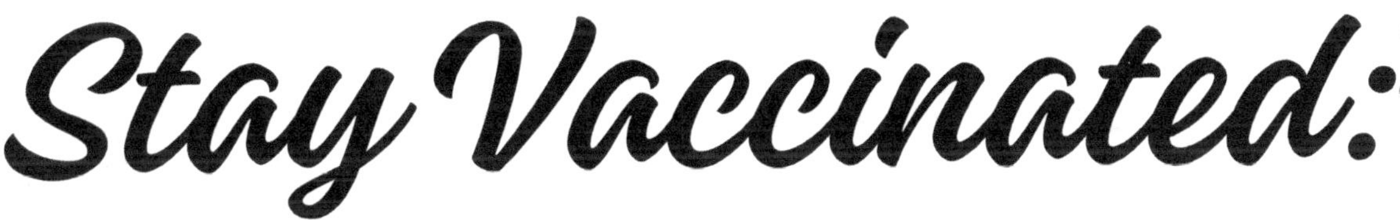

- Keep up with recommended vaccinations to protect against infectious diseases.
- Consult with your healthcare provider to ensure you are up-to-date on vaccines appropriate for your age and health status.

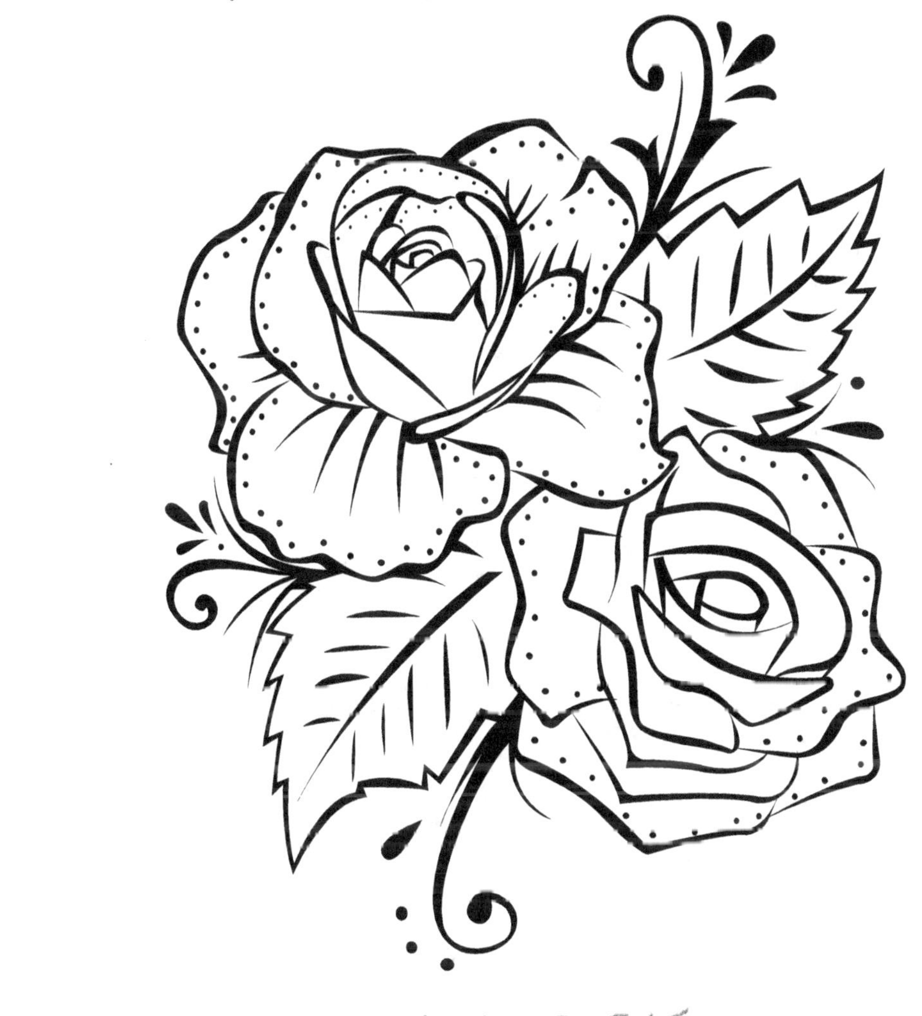

Mindful Breathing Exercises:

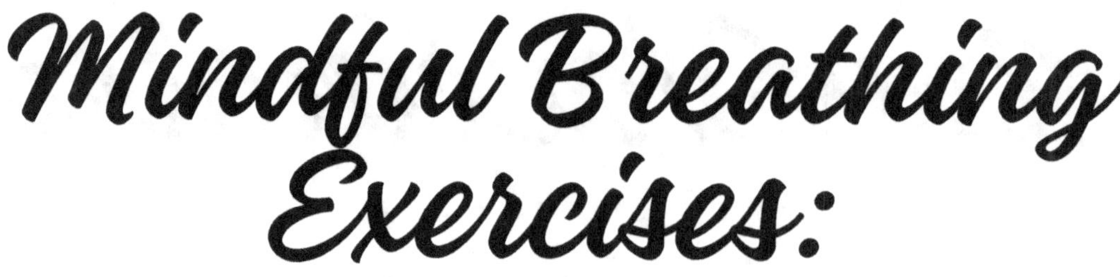

- Practice mindful breathing exercises to promote relaxation and reduce stress.
- Deep, intentional breathing can have positive effects on both physical and mental well-being.

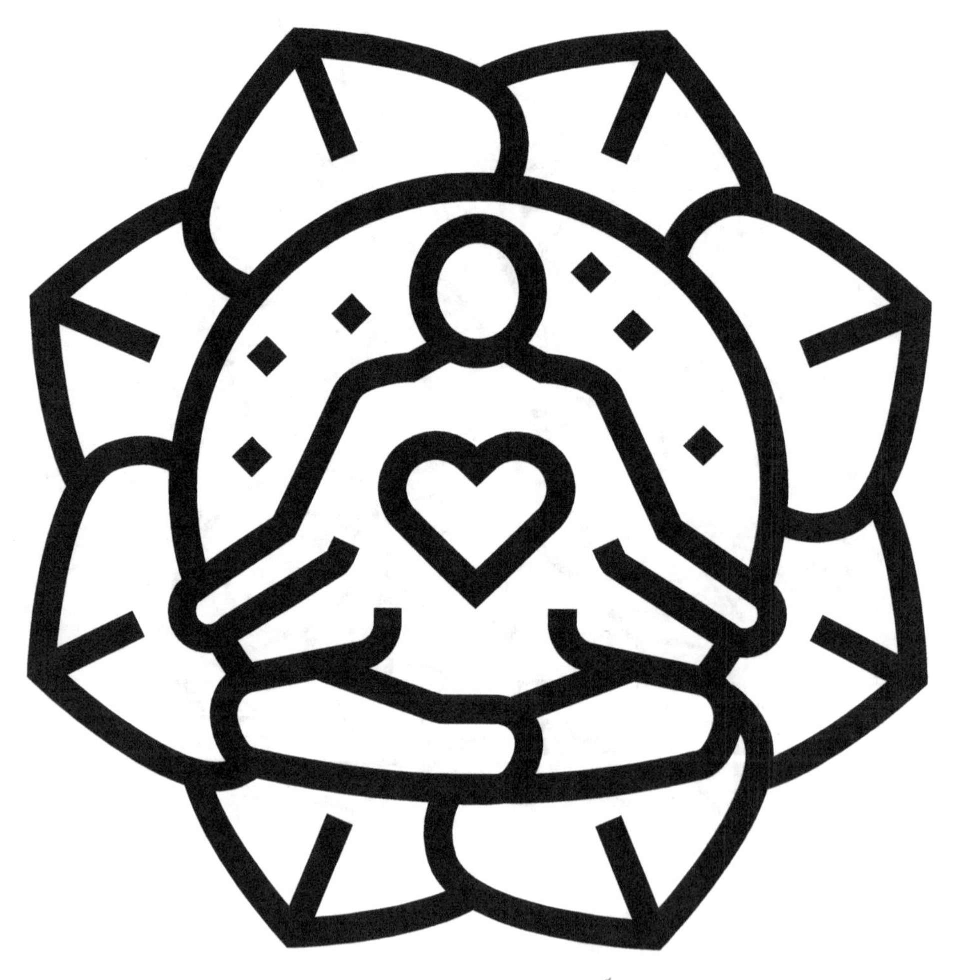

Explore Pet Therapy:

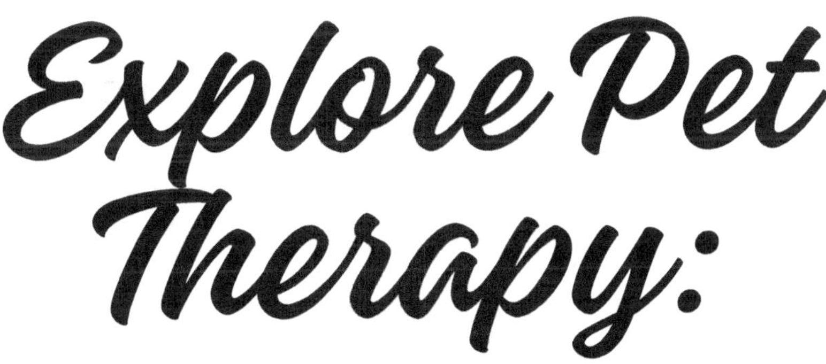

- Consider the companionship of pets, as they can provide emotional support and encourage physical activity.
- Walking a dog or spending time with a pet can contribute to a sense of purpose and joy.

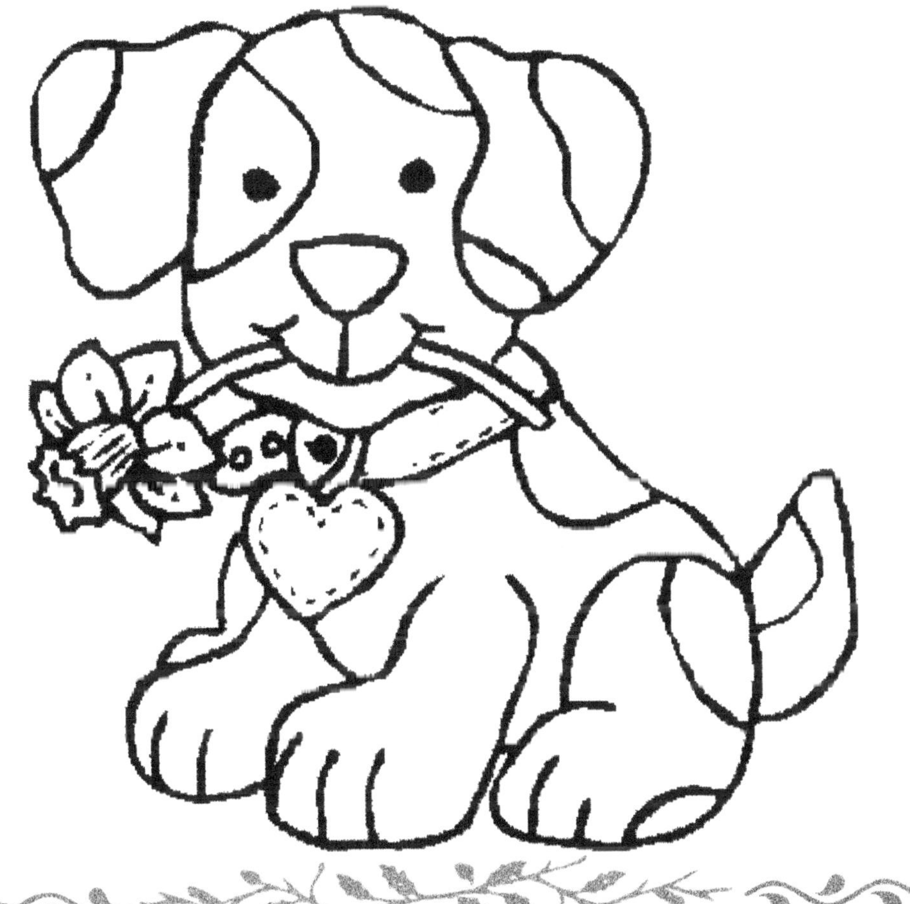

Engage in Intergenerational Activities:

- Connect with younger generations through activities that promote mutual understanding and enjoyment.
- Sharing experiences with younger family members or volunteering with youth organizations can bring new perspectives and energy.

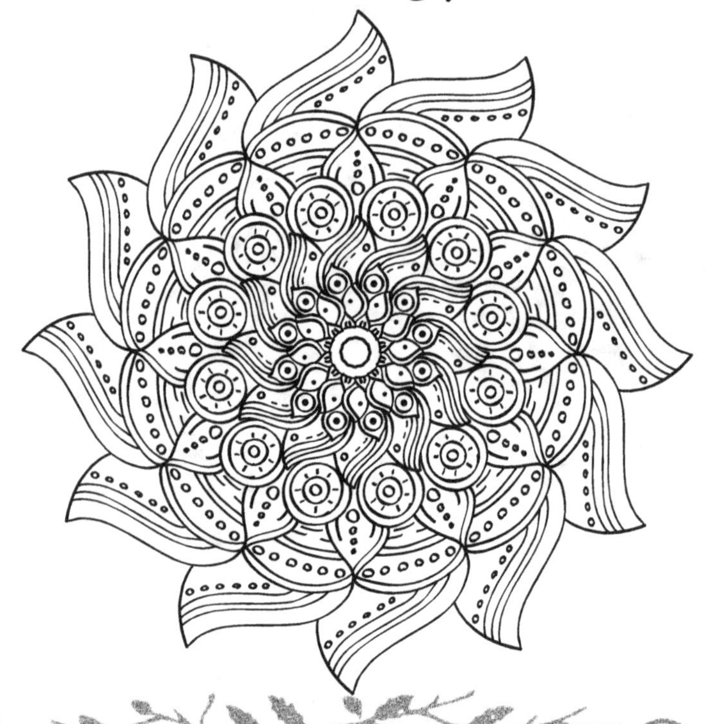

Maintain Strong Social Connections:

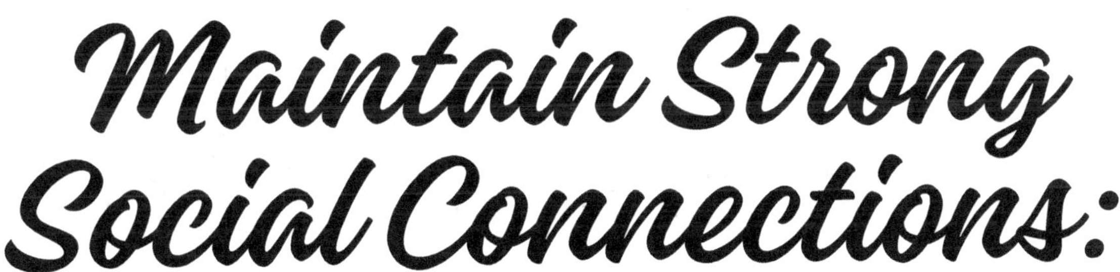

- Foster friendships and social connections to combat feelings of loneliness or isolation.
- Attend social events, join clubs, or participate in group activities to stay socially engaged.

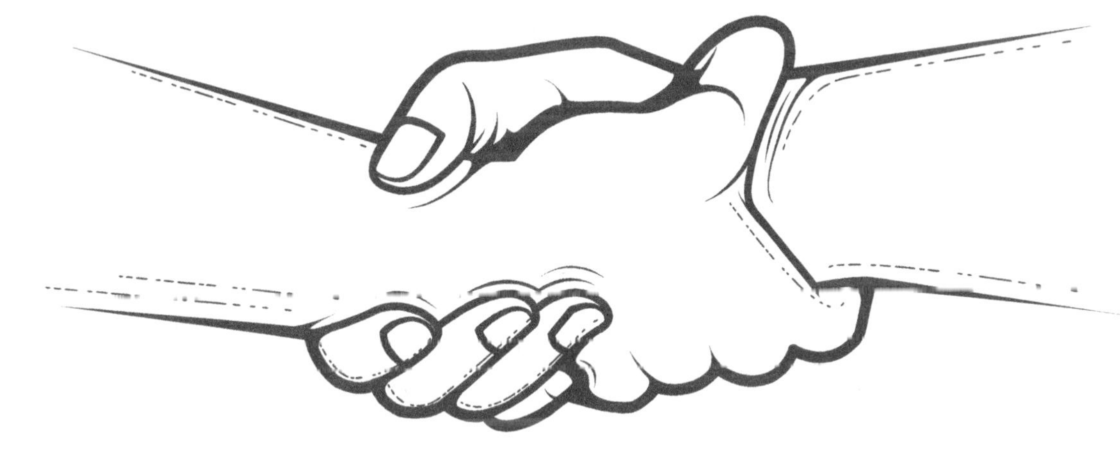

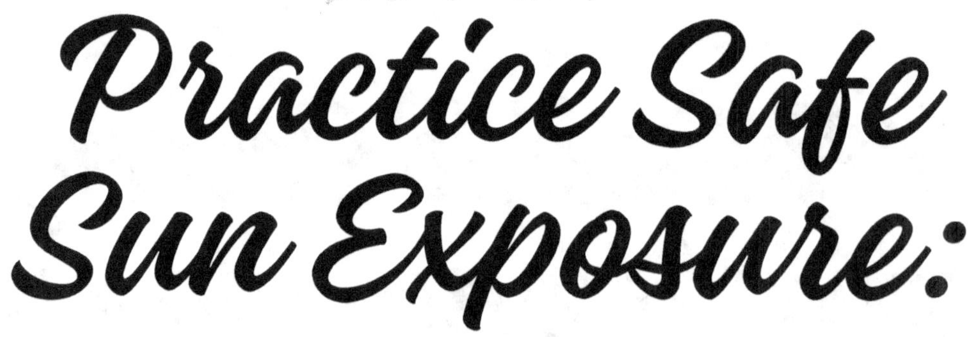

Practice Safe Sun Exposure:

- Enjoy the benefits of sunlight for vitamin D but protect your skin from harmful UV rays by using sunscreen and wearing protective clothing.
- Regular, moderate sun exposure can contribute to overall health and well-being.

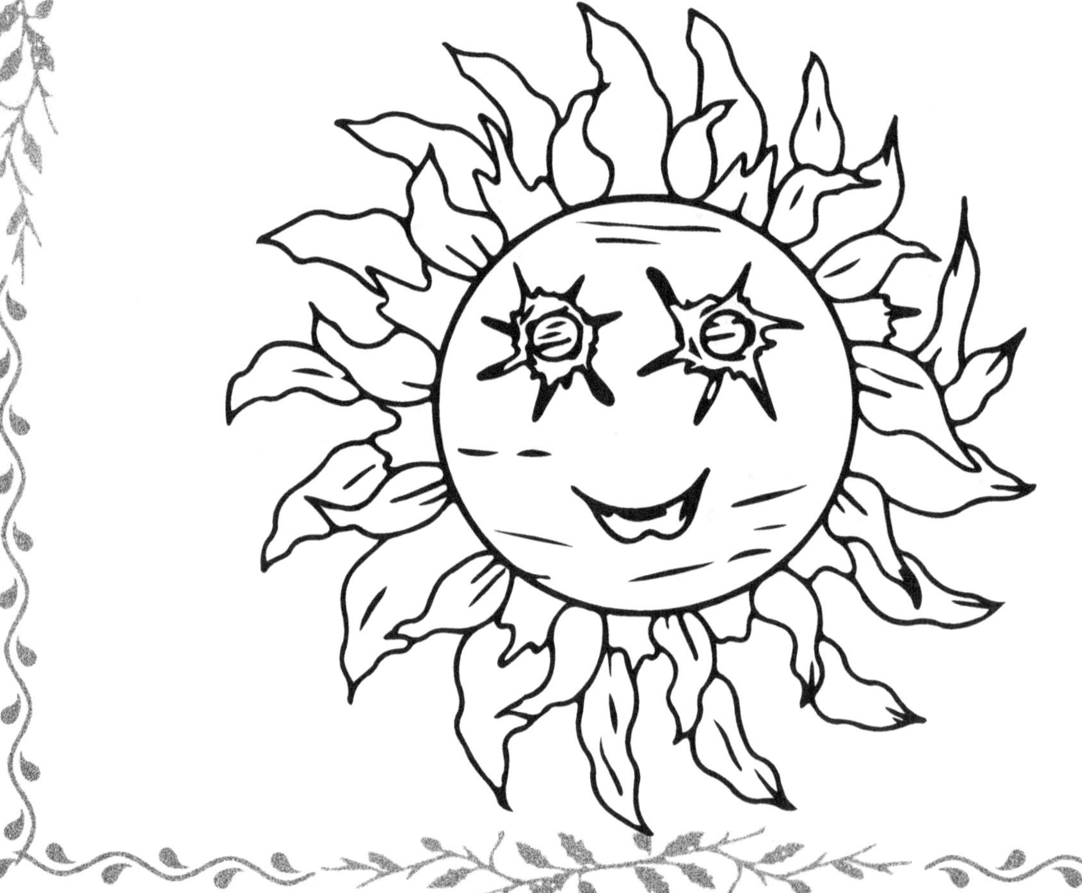

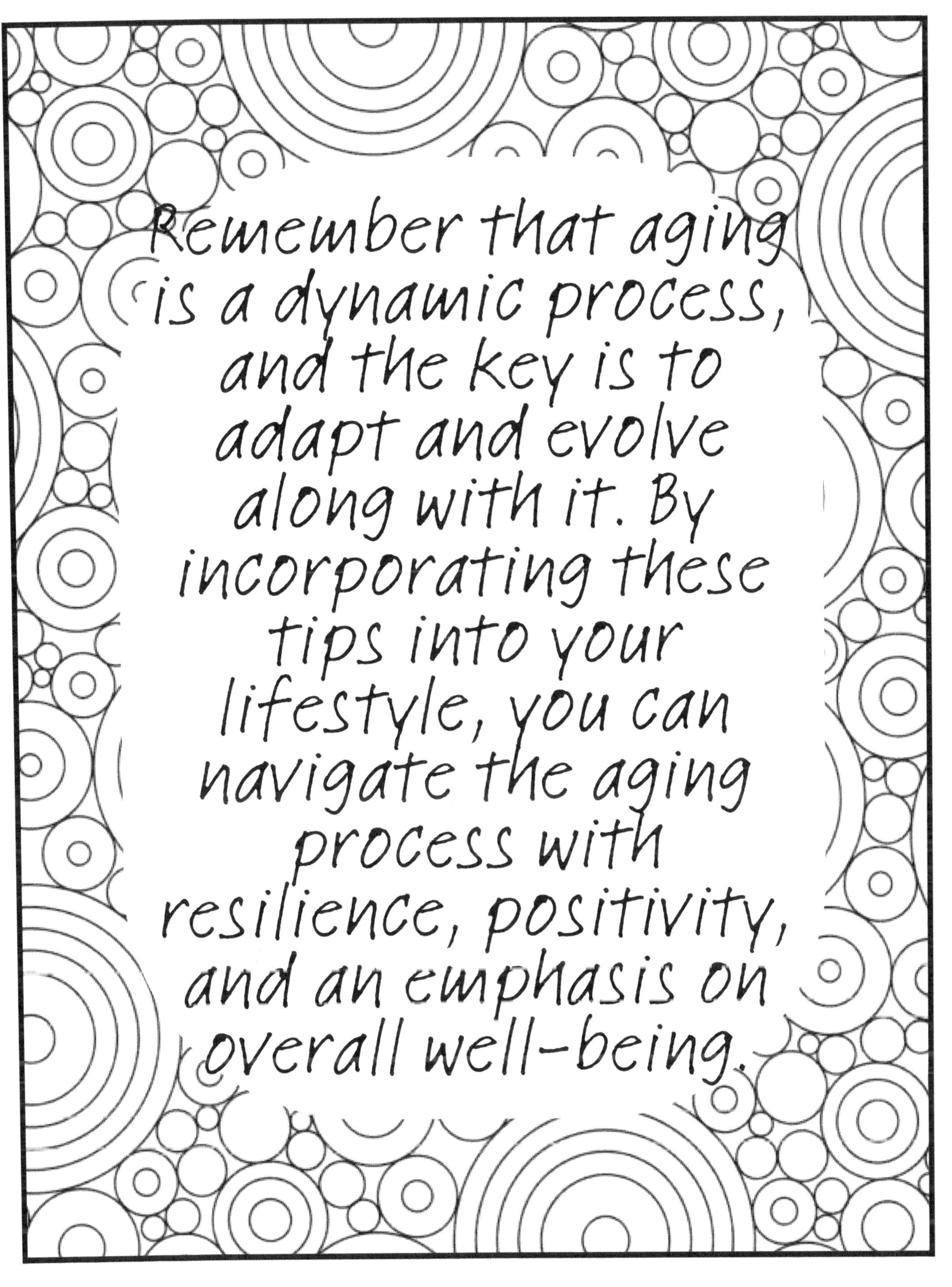

Remember that aging is a dynamic process, and the key is to adapt and evolve along with it. By incorporating these tips into your lifestyle, you can navigate the aging process with resilience, positivity, and an emphasis on overall well-being.

Explore Gentle Therapeutic Exercises:

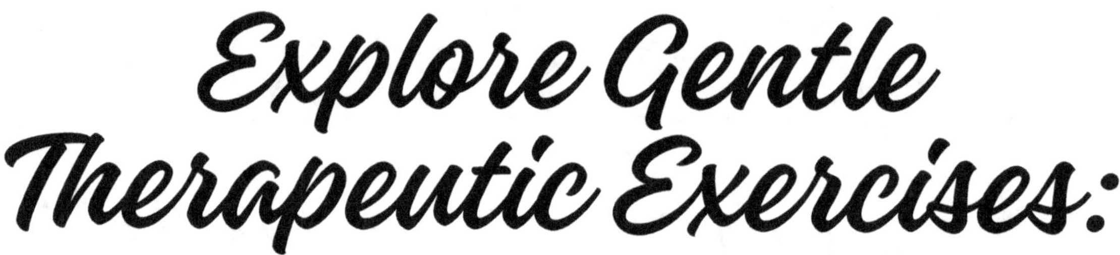

- Investigate therapeutic exercises tailored to your specific needs, such as water aerobics or gentle yoga.
- These activities can improve mobility, flexibility, and overall physical function.

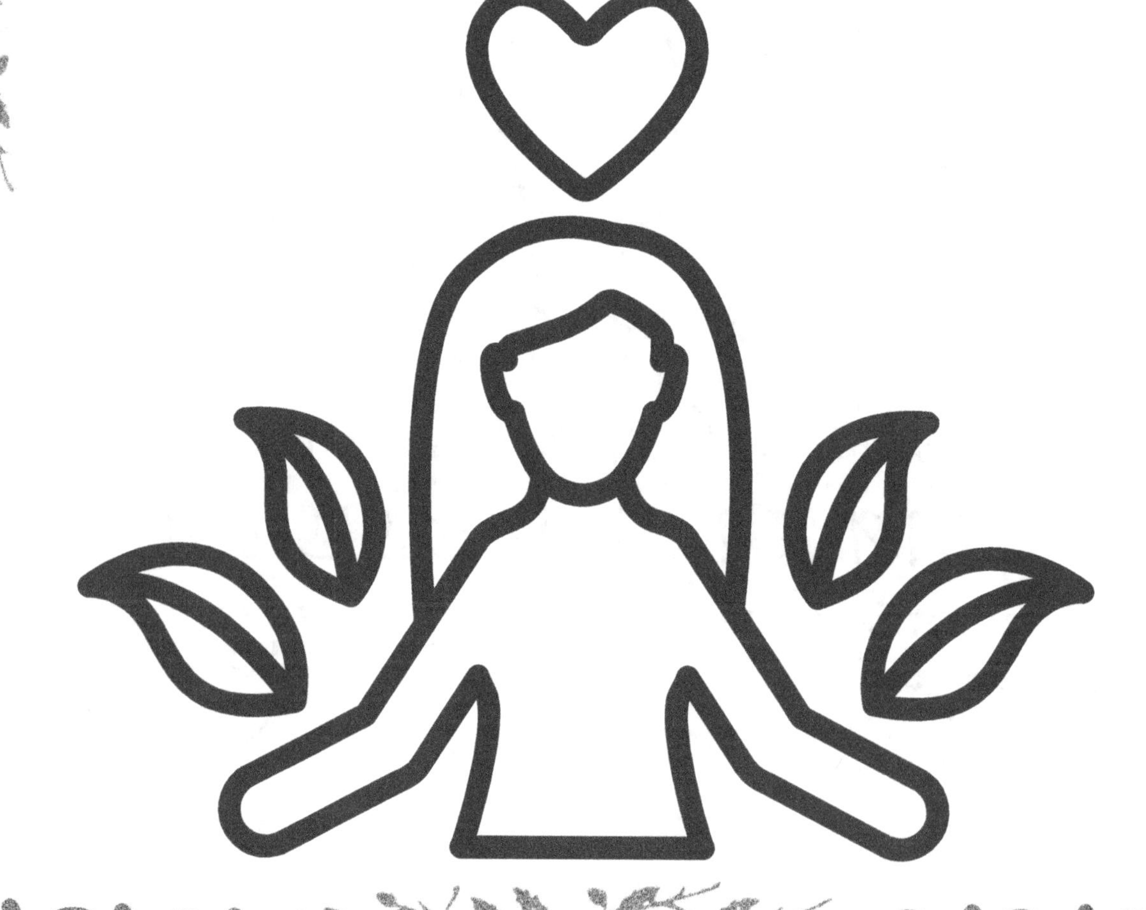

Contribute to Your Community:

- Engage in community service or volunteer work to stay active, connected, and make a positive impact.
- Contributing to the well-being of others can bring a sense of fulfillment and purpose.

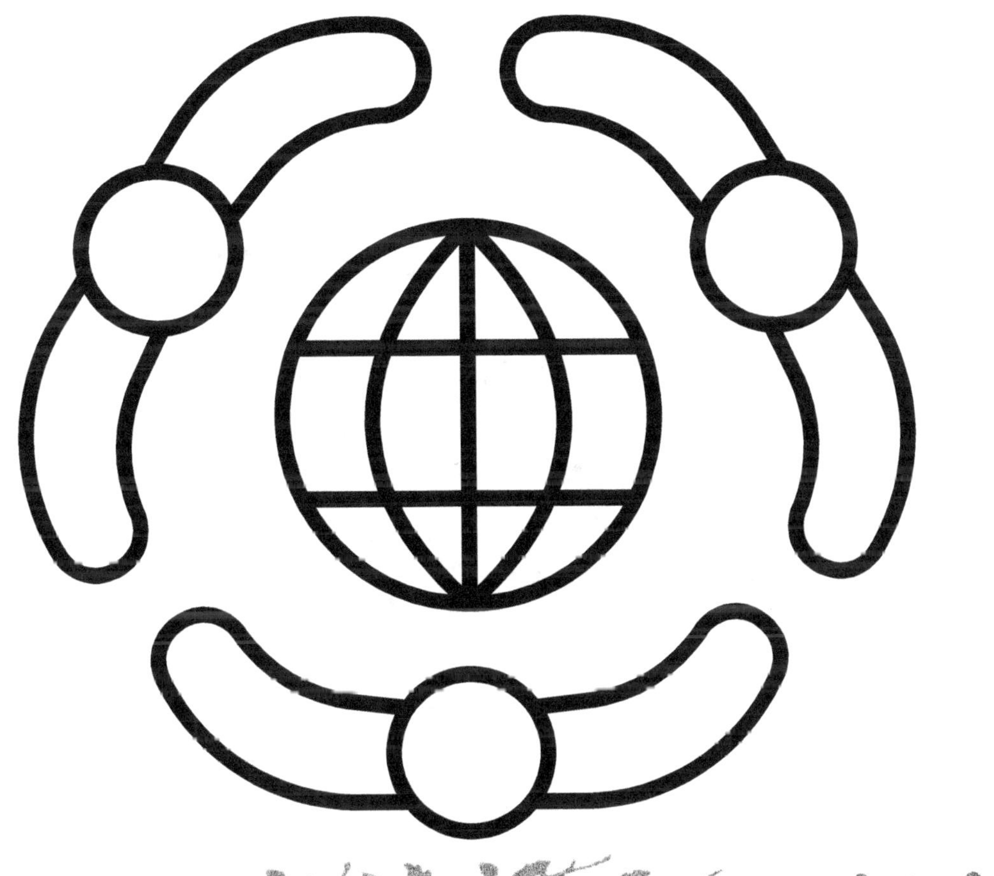

Manage Chronic Conditions Proactively:

- If you have chronic health conditions, work closely with your healthcare team to manage them effectively.
- Regular monitoring and proactive management can help you maintain a good quality of life.

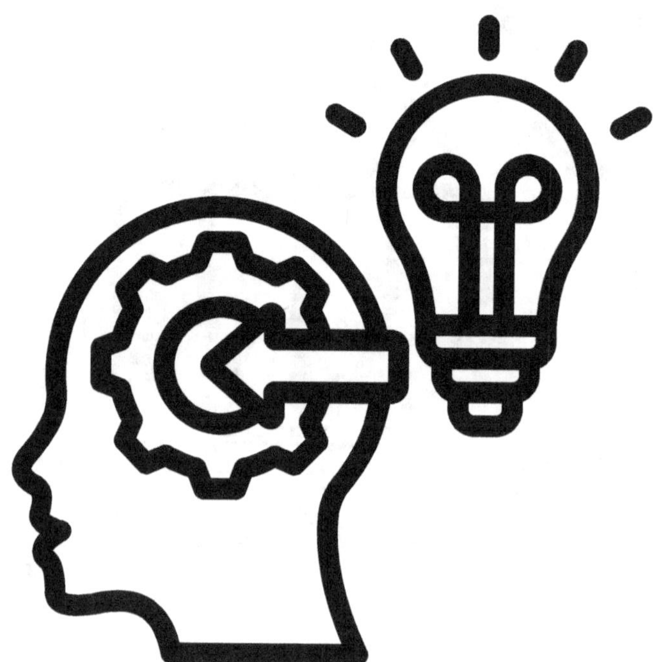

Regular Dental Check-ups:

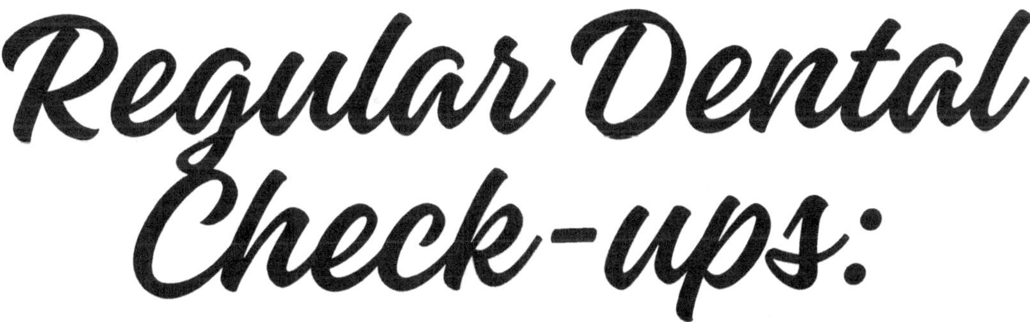

- Schedule routine dental check-ups and cleanings to maintain oral health.
- Good oral hygiene contributes not only to dental health but also to overall well-being.

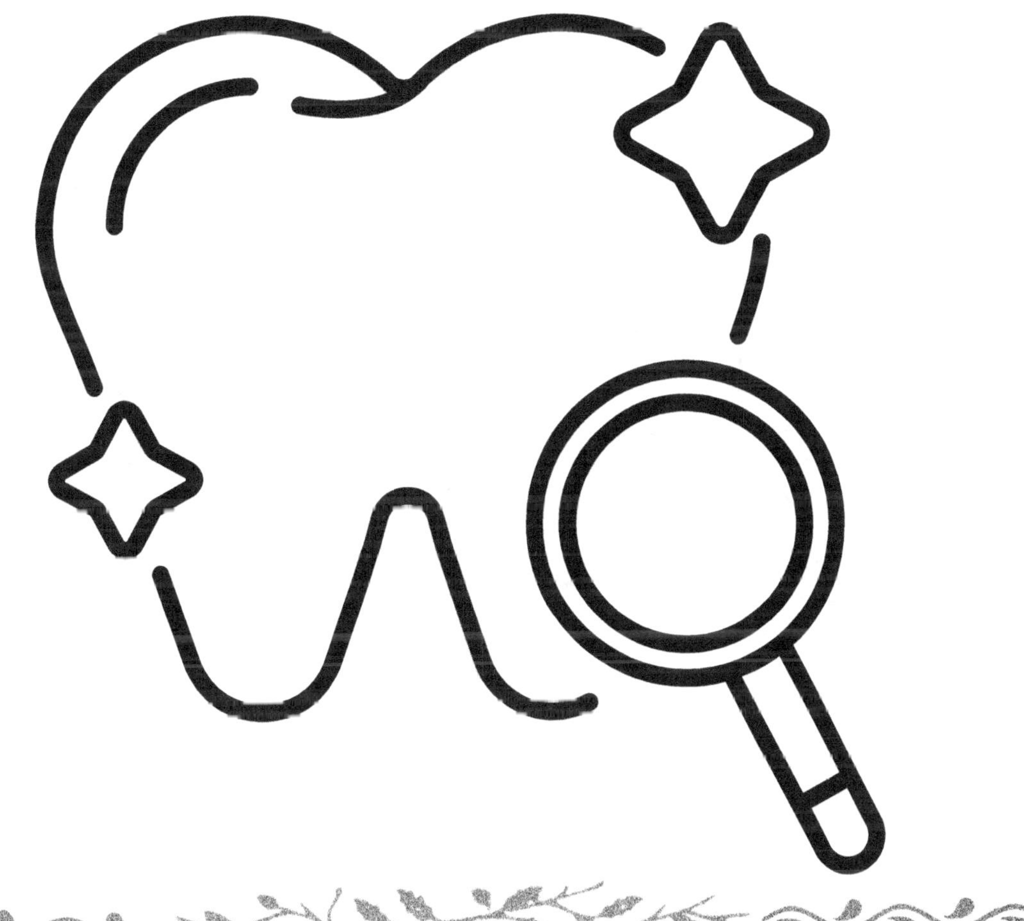

Adopt a Holistic Approach:

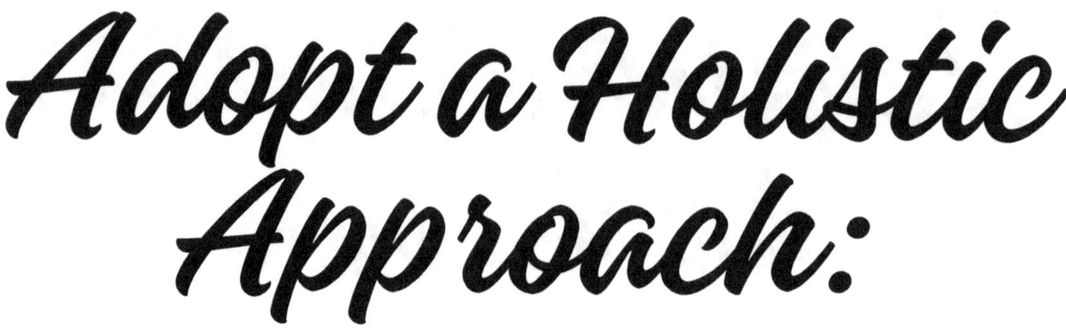

- Embrace a holistic approach to health that considers the interconnectedness of physical, mental, and emotional well-being.
- Addressing multiple aspects of health can lead to a more balanced and fulfilling life.

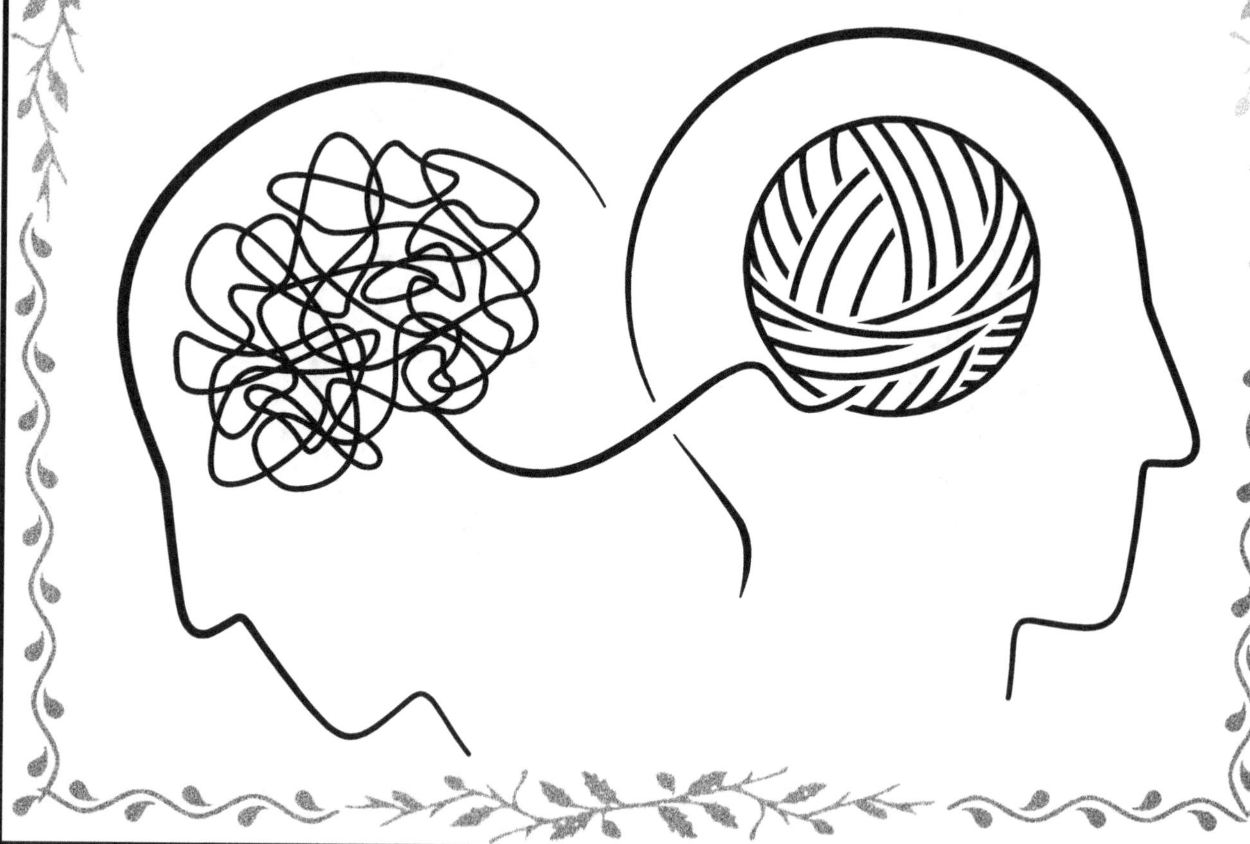

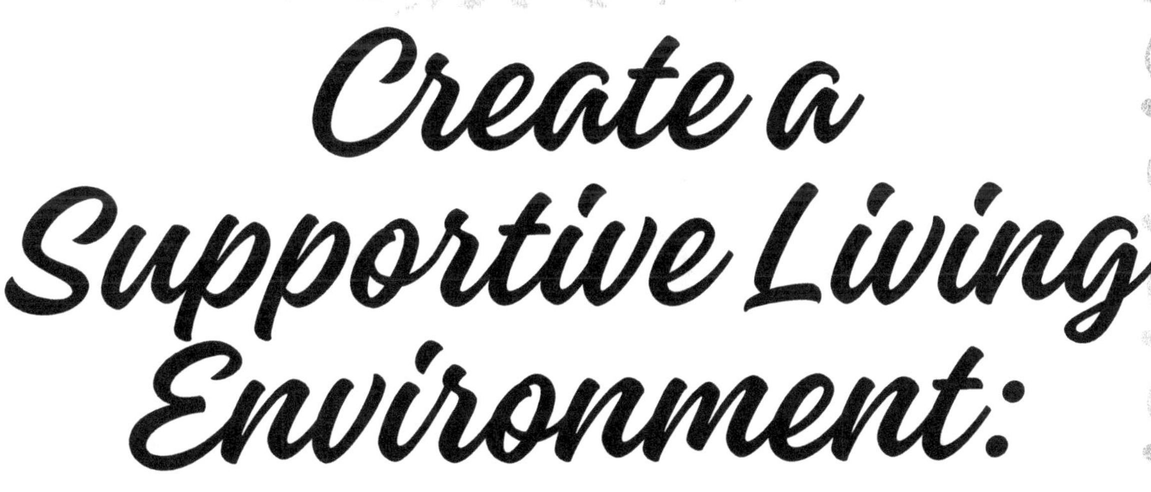

Create a Supportive Living Environment:

- Ensure your living environment is conducive to your well-being, considering factors like lighting, safety, and accessibility.
- Make adjustments as needed to create a comfortable and supportive space.

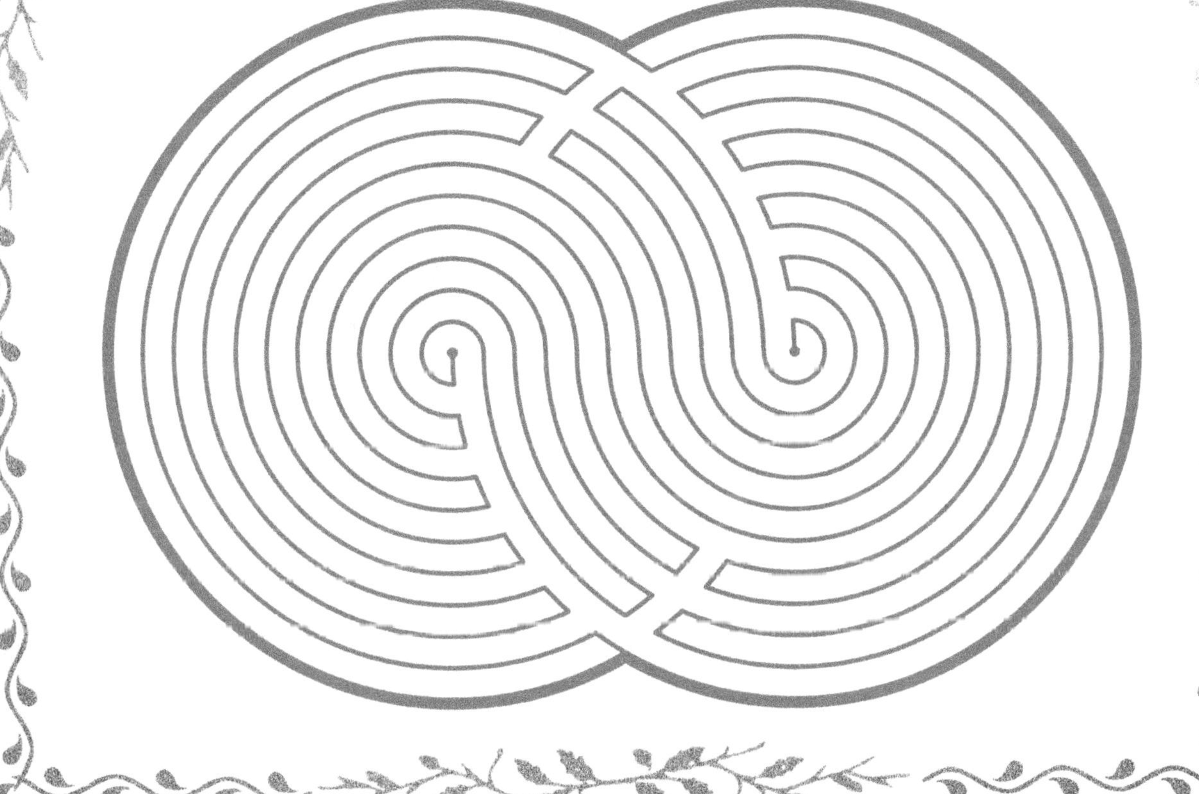

Hygiene and Skin Care:

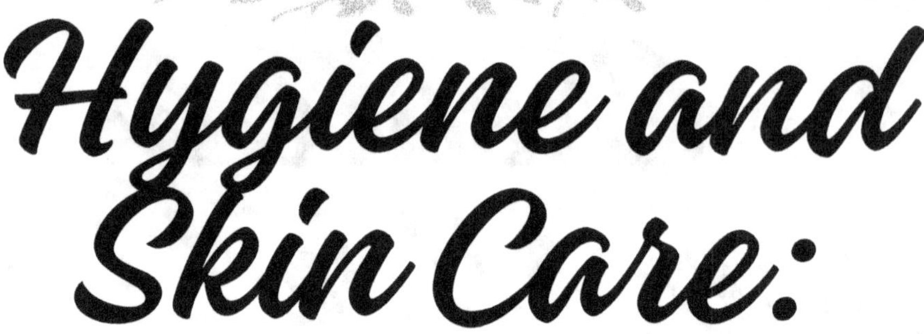

- Maintain good hygiene practices to prevent infections and promote overall health.
- Pay attention to skin care by using moisturizers and addressing any skin conditions promptly.

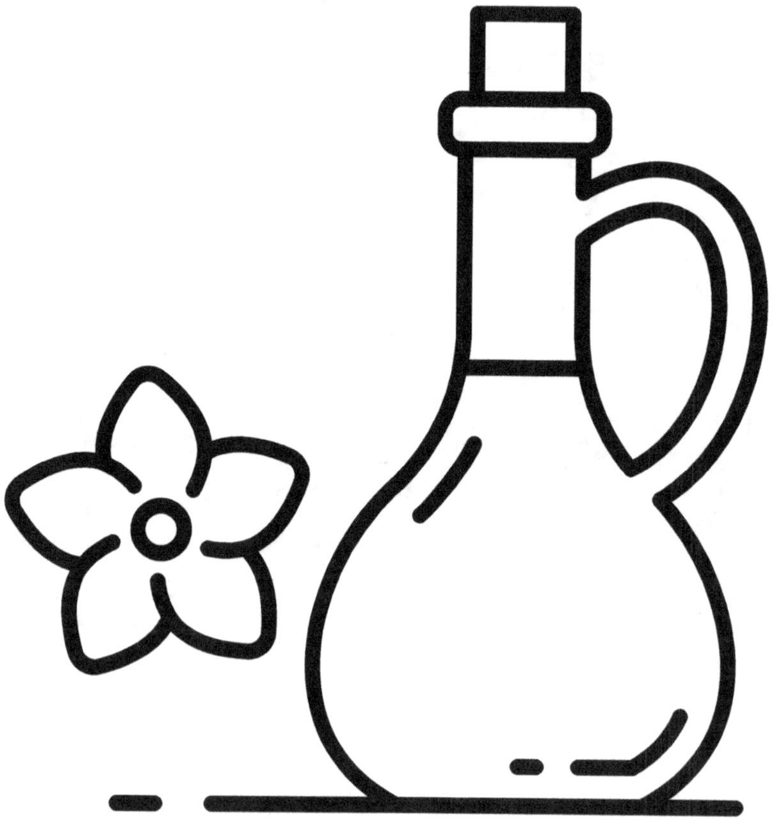

Cultivate a Healthy Sleep Routine:

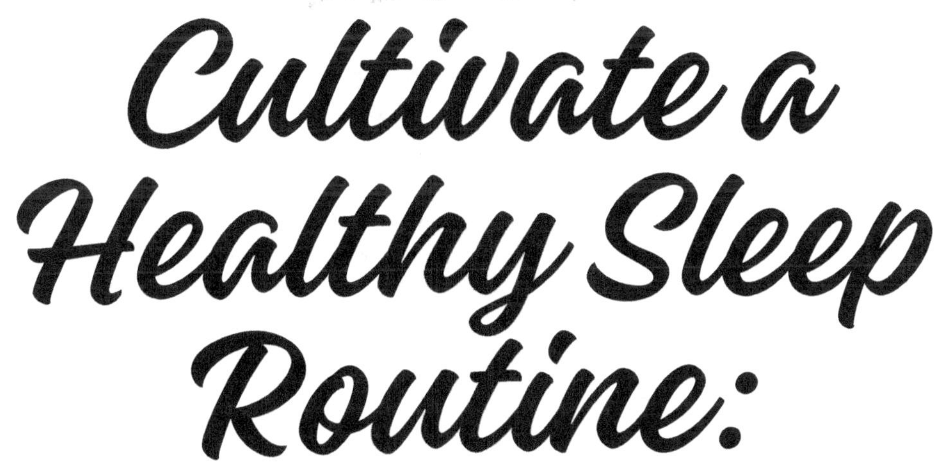

- Prioritize sufficient and restful sleep by establishing a consistent sleep routine.
- Create a comfortable sleep environment with proper bedding and minimal disturbances.

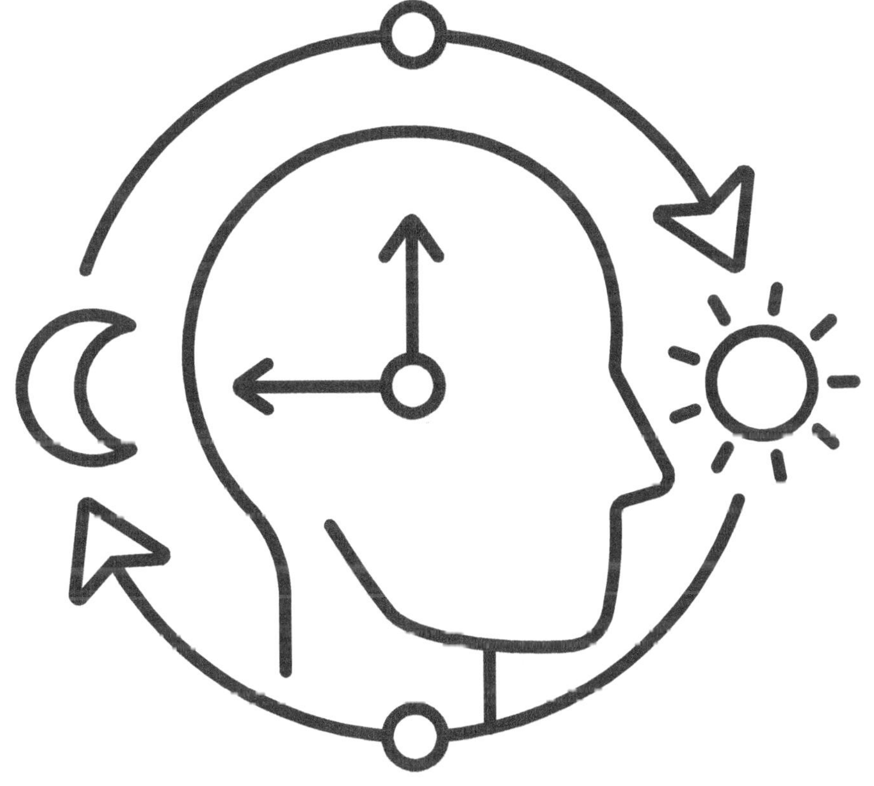

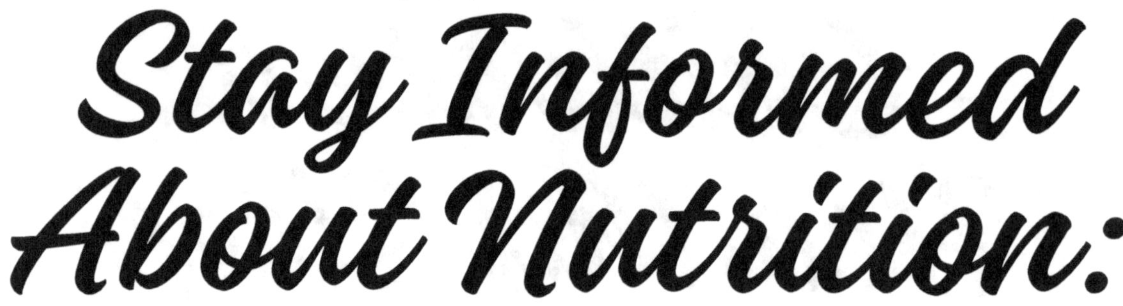

Stay Informed About Nutrition:

- Stay updated on nutritional needs specific to your age and health condition.
- Consult with a registered dietitian to ensure your diet supports your overall well-being.

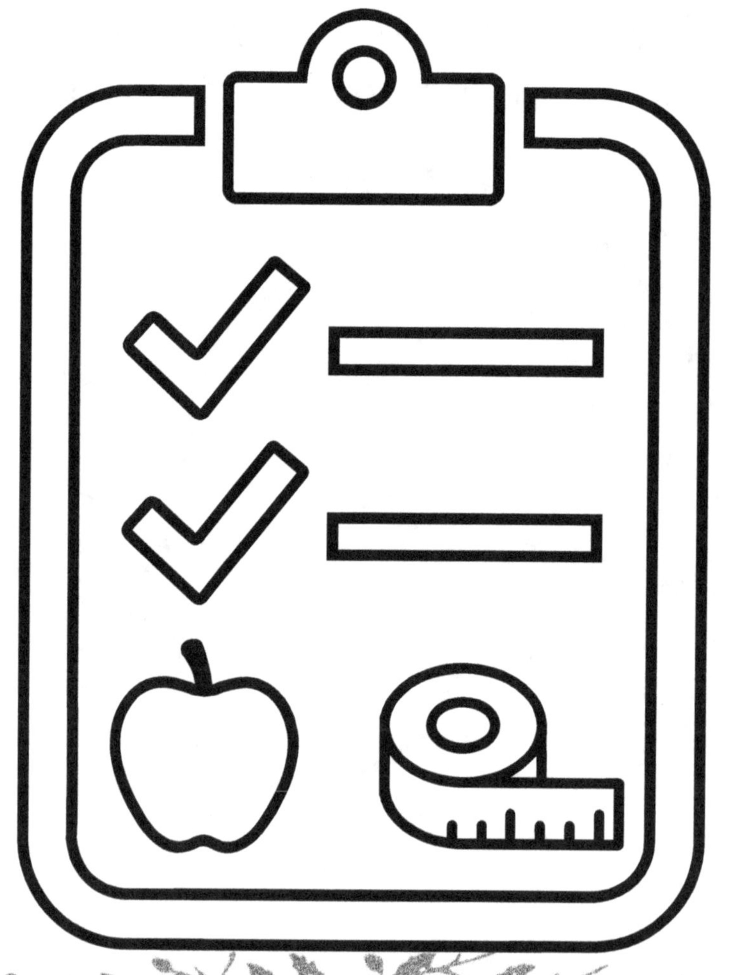

Mindfulness Meditation:

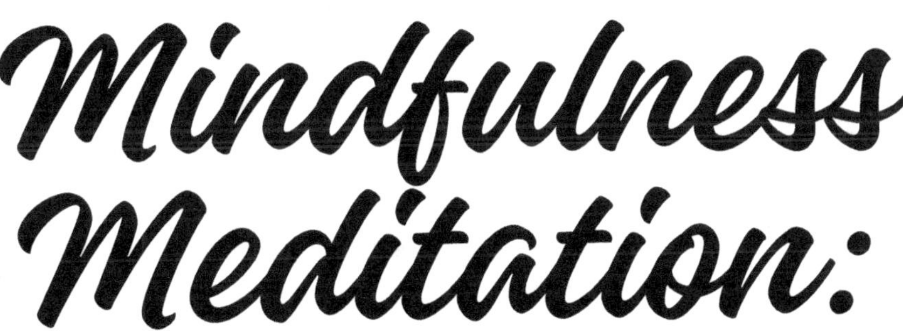

- Incorporate mindfulness meditation into your daily routine to promote relaxation and reduce stress.
- Mindfulness practices can contribute to mental clarity and emotional resilience.

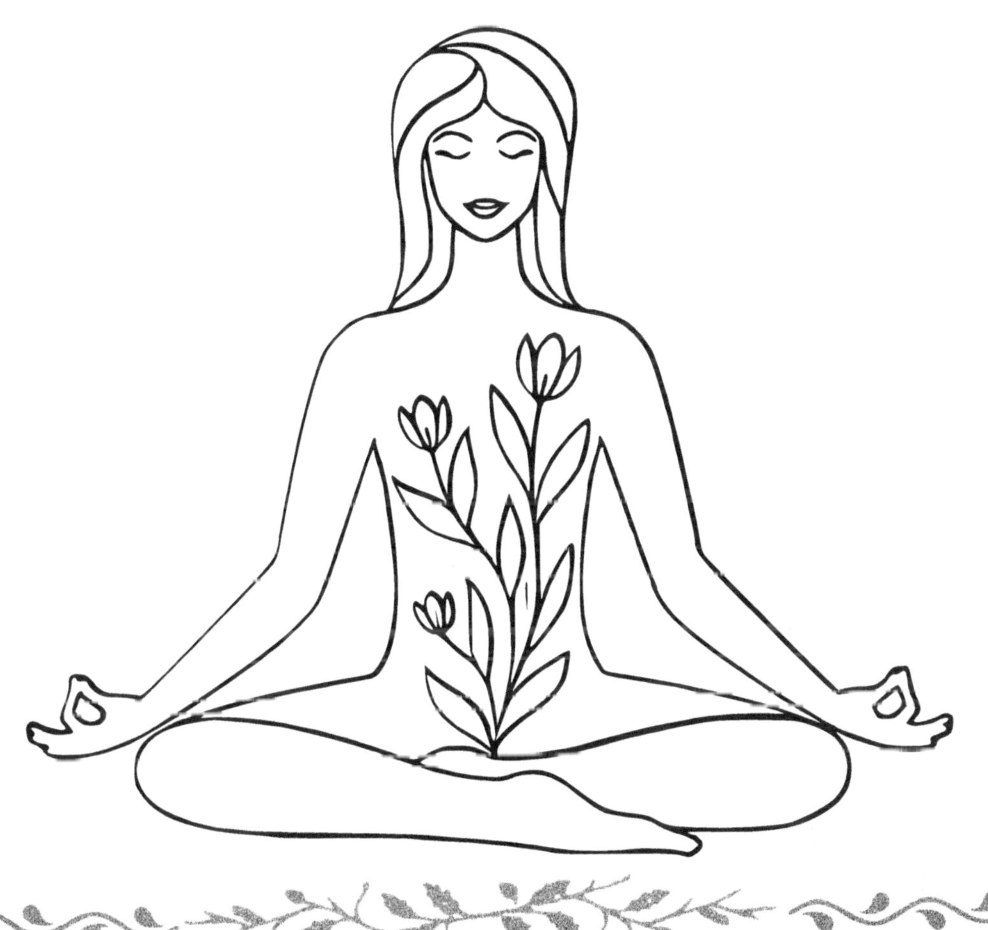

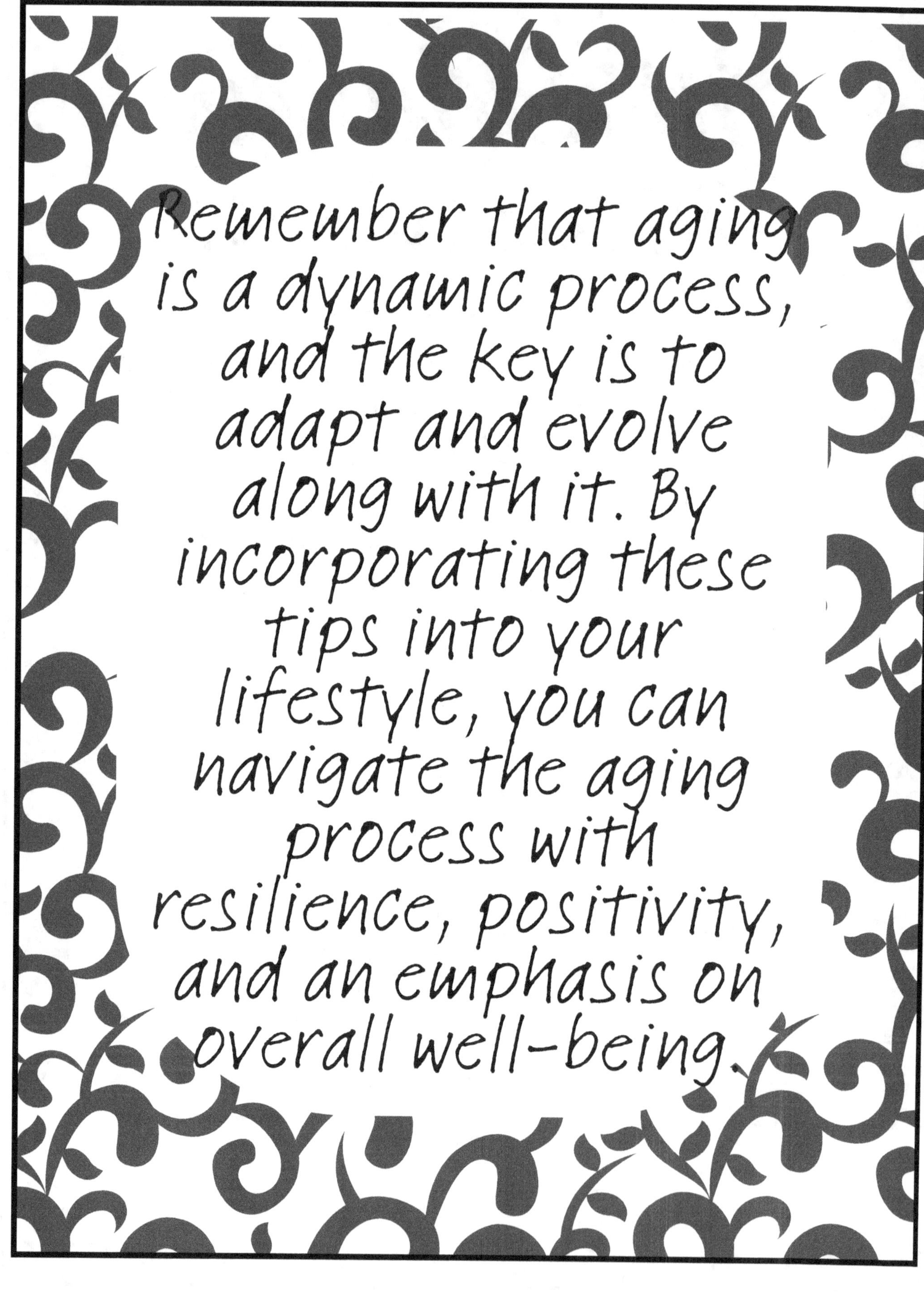

Remember that aging is a dynamic process, and the key is to adapt and evolve along with it. By incorporating these tips into your lifestyle, you can navigate the aging process with resilience, positivity, and an emphasis on overall well-being.

Invest in Ergonomic Solutions:

- Consider ergonomic solutions for your living and workspaces to reduce physical strain.
- Use supportive chairs, pillows, or keyboard stands to enhance comfort.

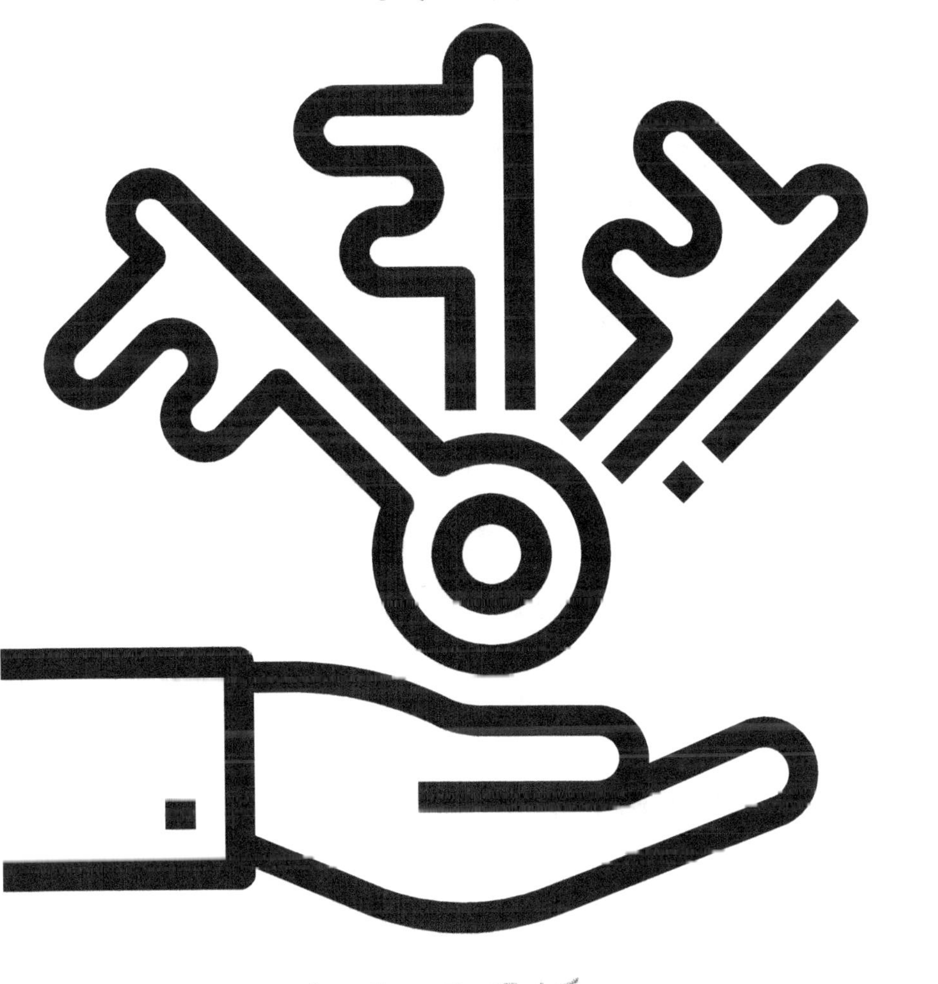

Express Yourself Creatively:

- Explore creative outlets such as painting, writing, or music to express yourself.
- Engaging in artistic activities can provide a sense of accomplishment and joy.

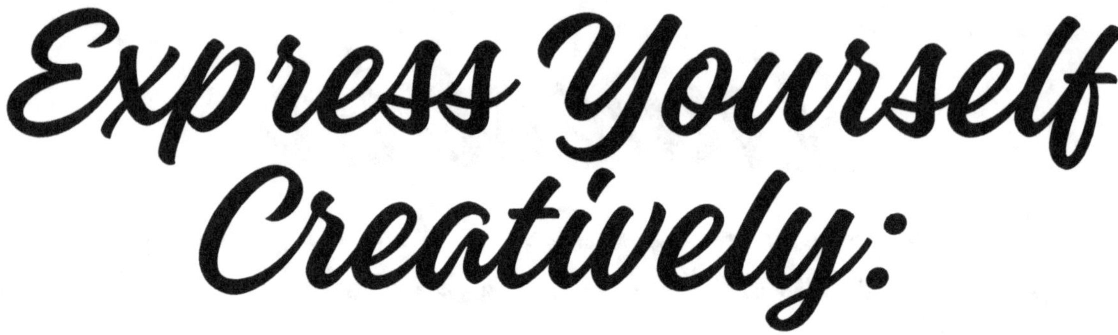

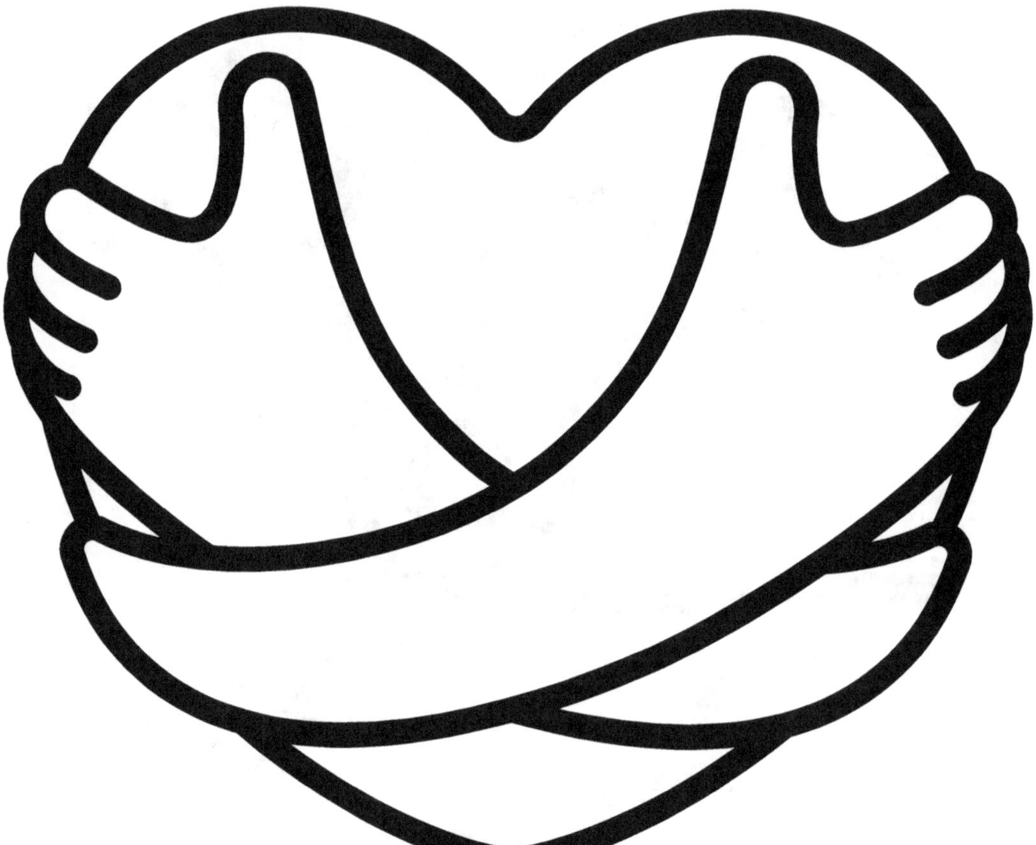

Stay Adaptable:

- Embrace adaptability in the face of changing circumstances.
- Be open to trying new approaches and solutions to overcome challenges.

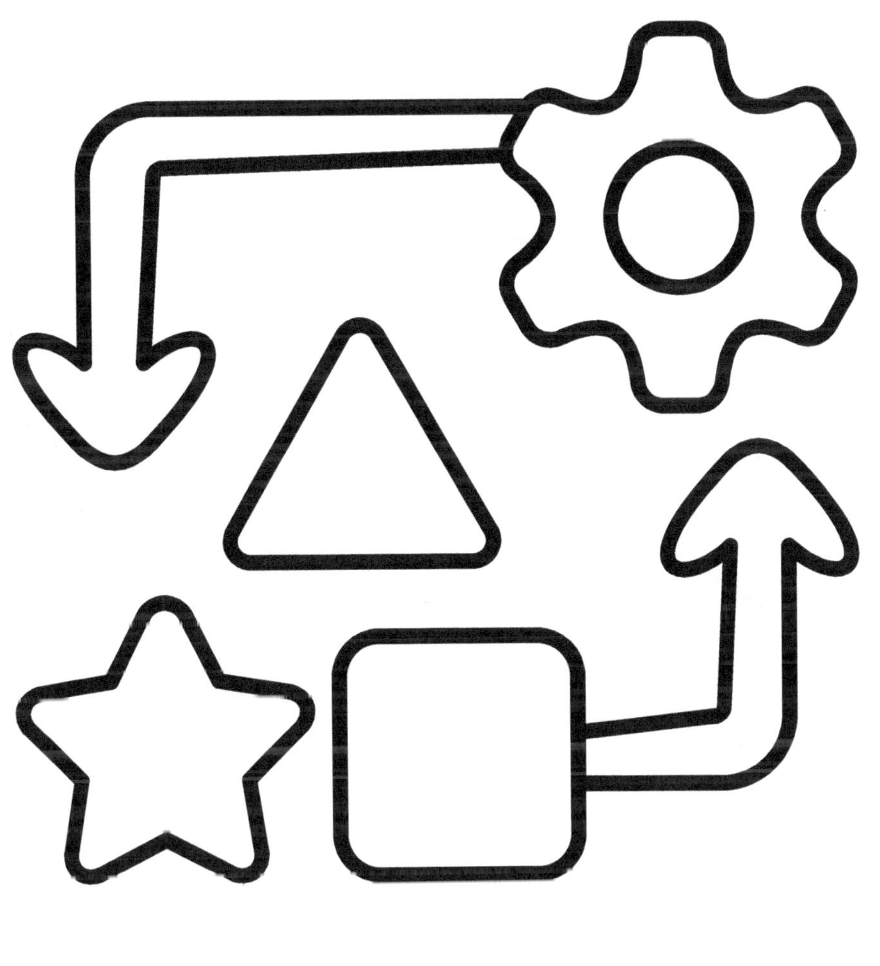

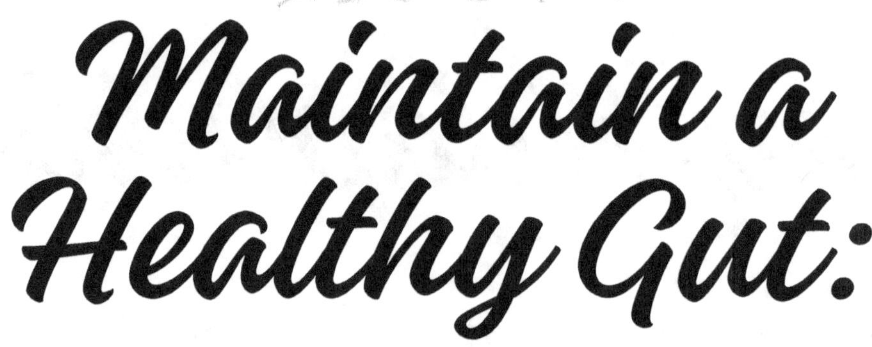

Maintain a Healthy Gut:

- Support digestive health by incorporating fiber-rich foods and probiotics into your diet.
- A healthy gut contributes to overall immune function and well-being.

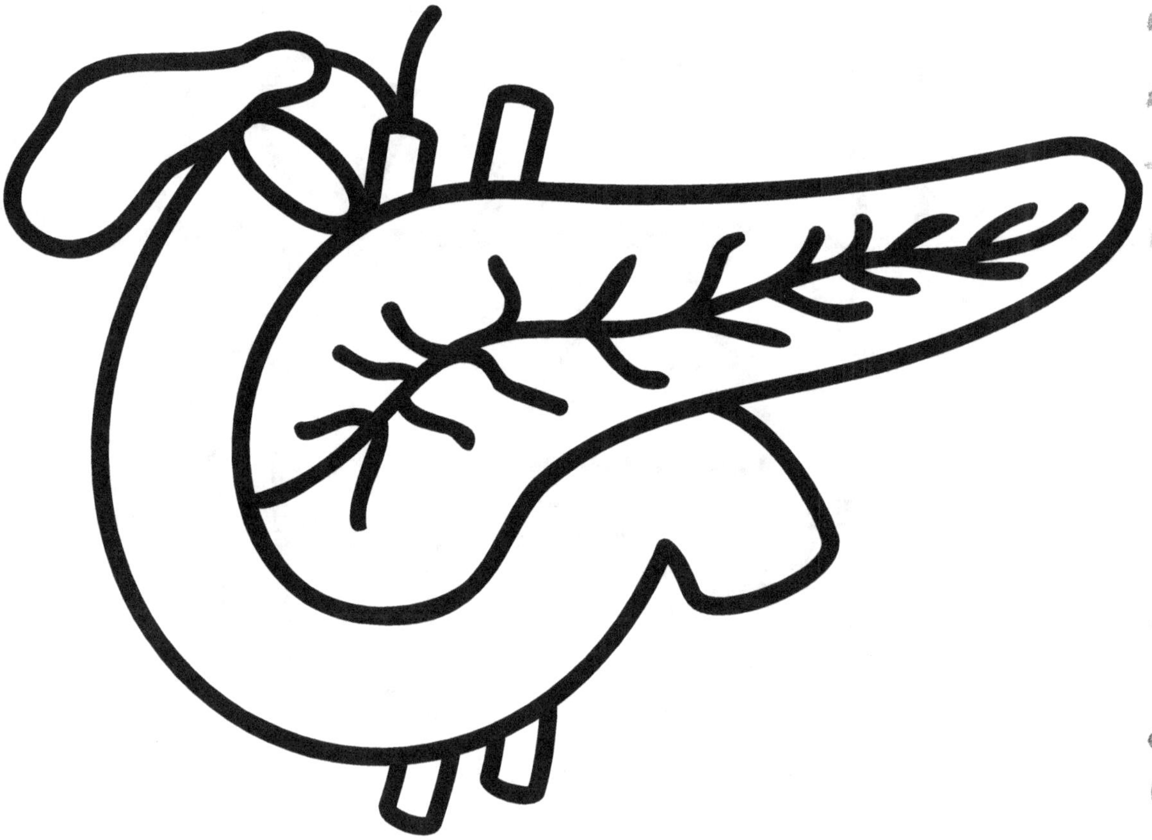

Set Realistic Goals:

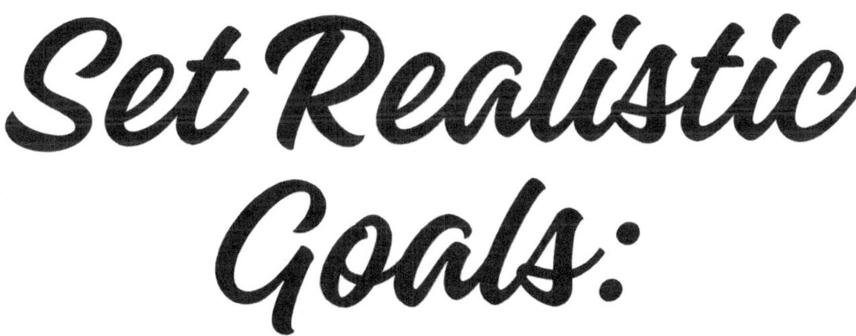

- Establish realistic and achievable goals for yourself, both short-term and long-term.
- Celebrate progress and adjust goals as needed to align with your capabilities.

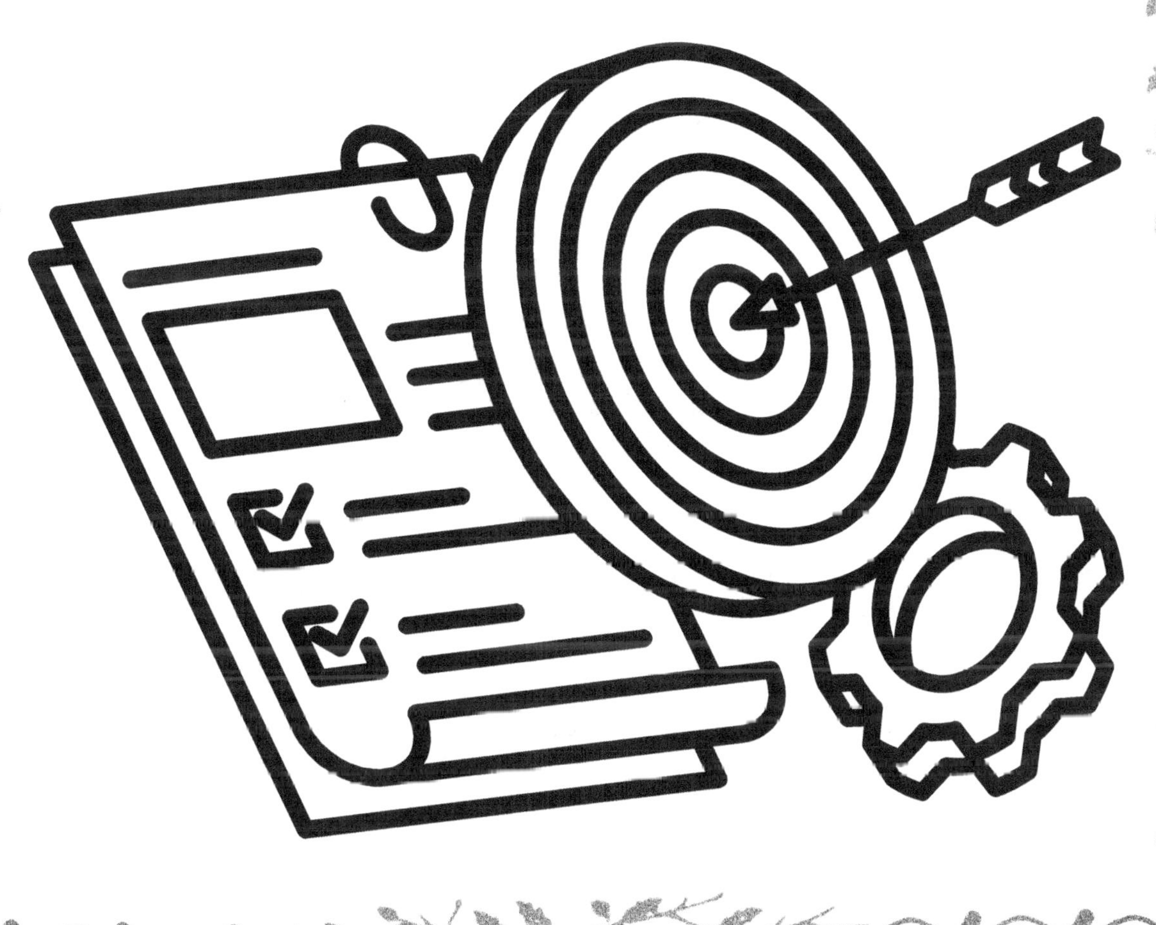

Embrace Technology for Learning:

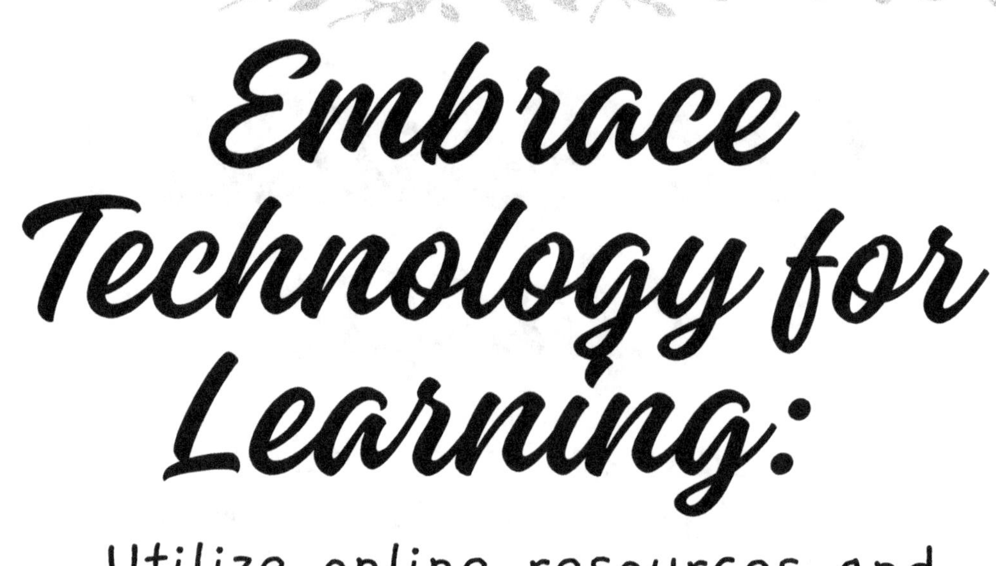

- Utilize online resources and courses to continue learning and staying mentally active.
- Online platforms offer a wealth of information and opportunities for skill development.

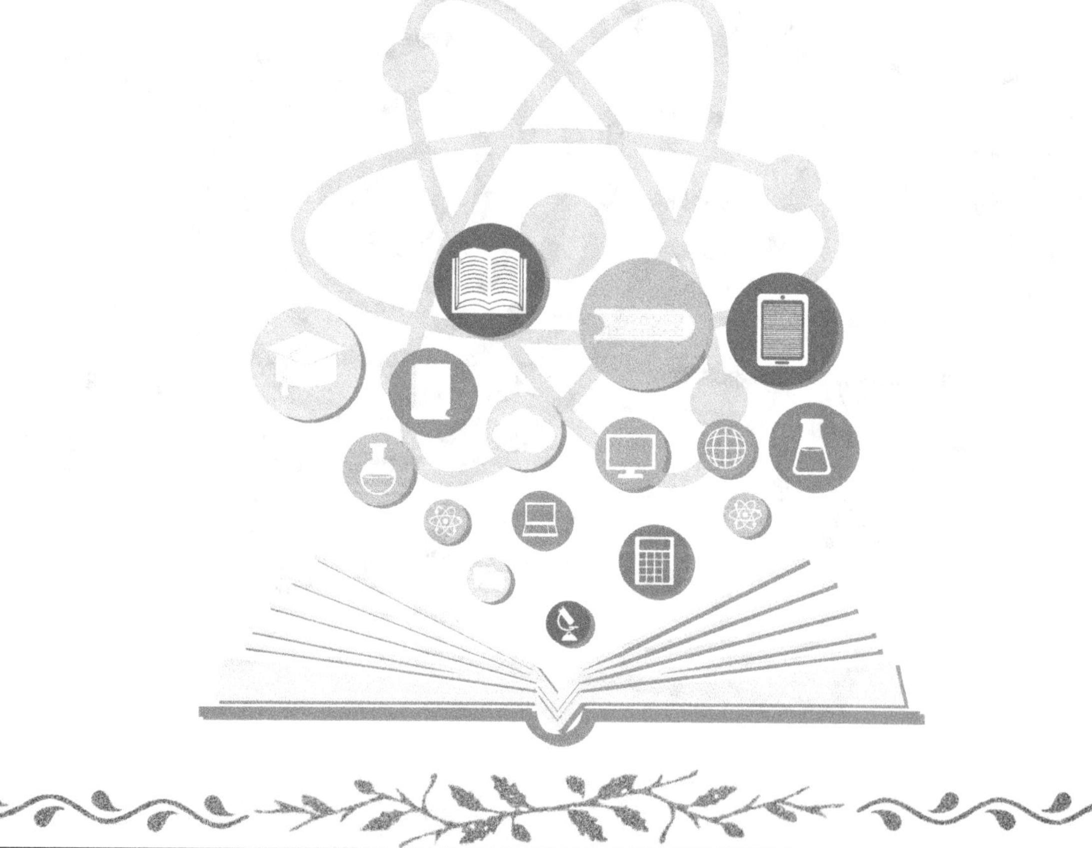

Stay Financially Savvy:

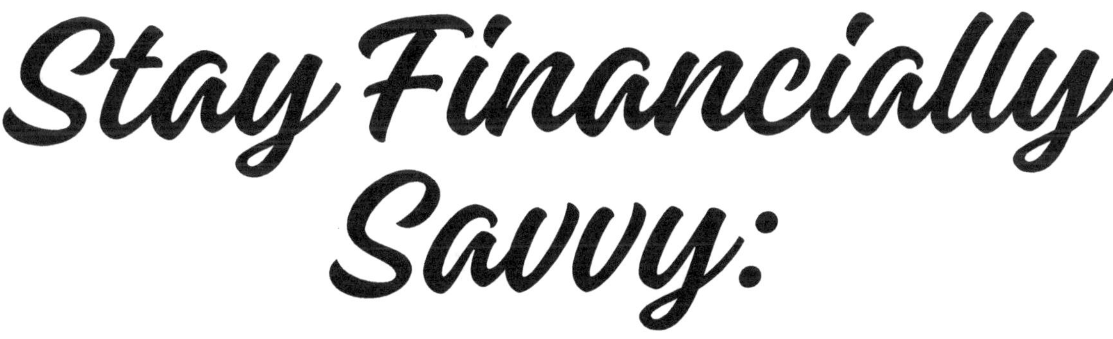

- Stay informed about financial planning and manage resources wisely.
- Work with financial advisors to ensure a secure and comfortable retirement.

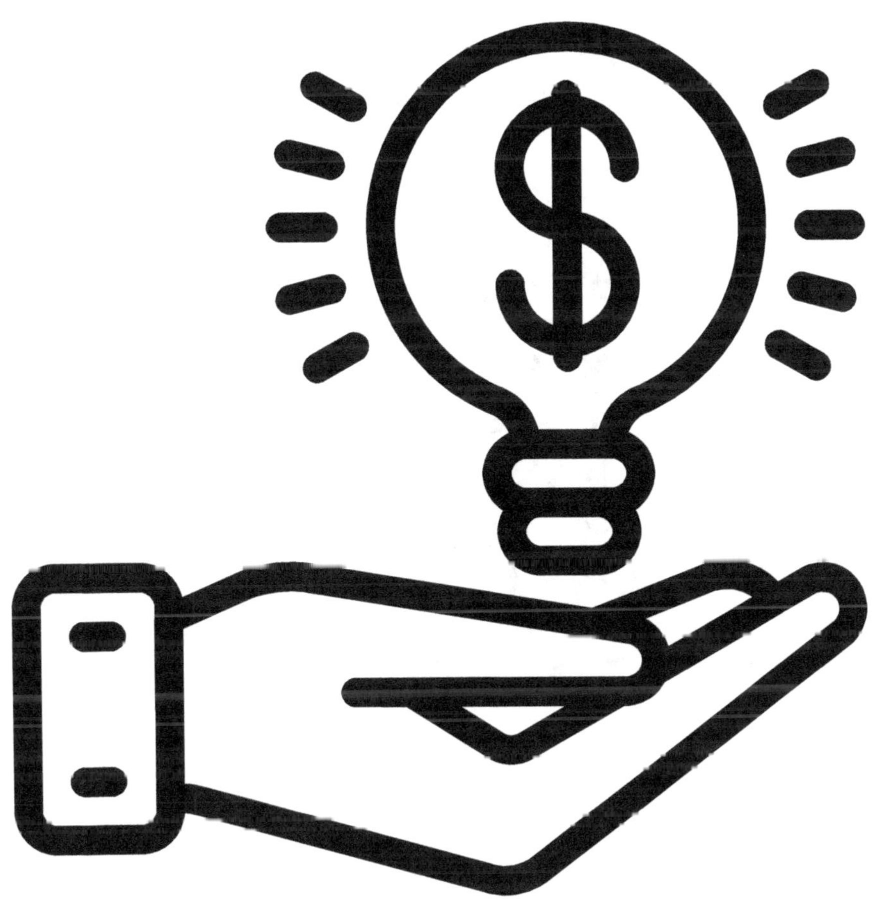

Practice Patience and Self-Compassion:

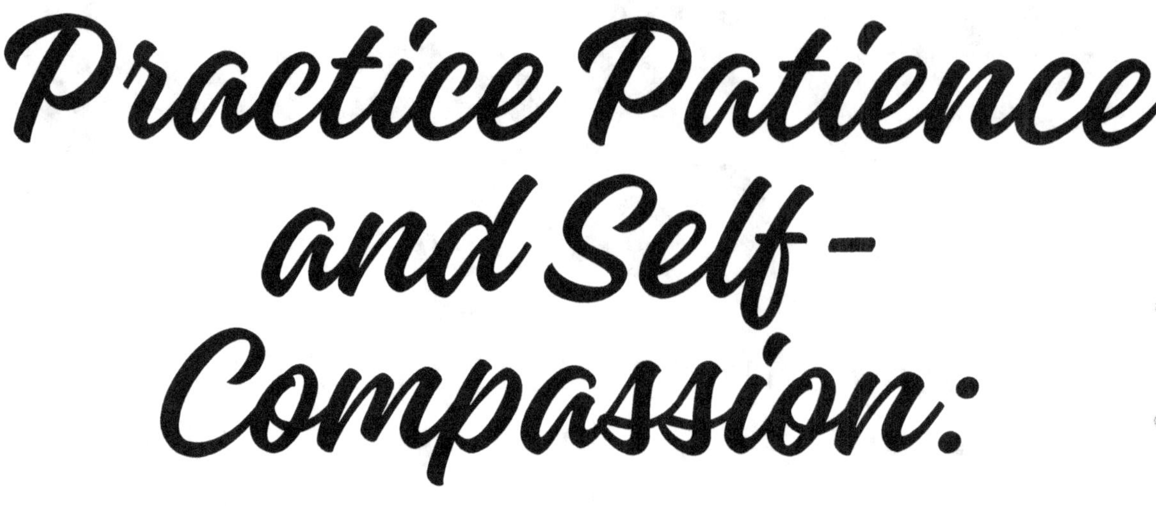

- Be patient with yourself as you navigate changes and challenges.
- Practice self-compassion and acknowledge that it's okay to ask for help when needed.

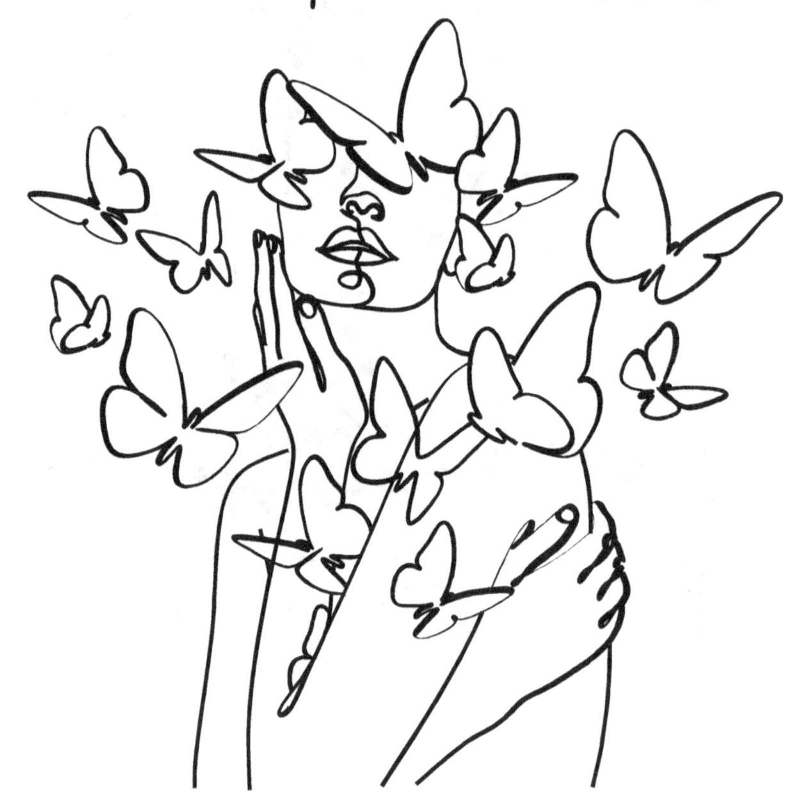

Enjoy the Outdoors:

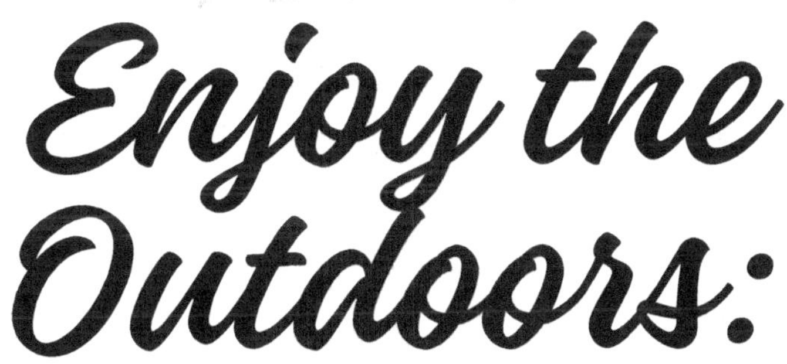

- Spend time outdoors enjoying nature and sunlight.
- Activities like walking, gardening, or simply being in nature can have positive effects on both physical and mental health.

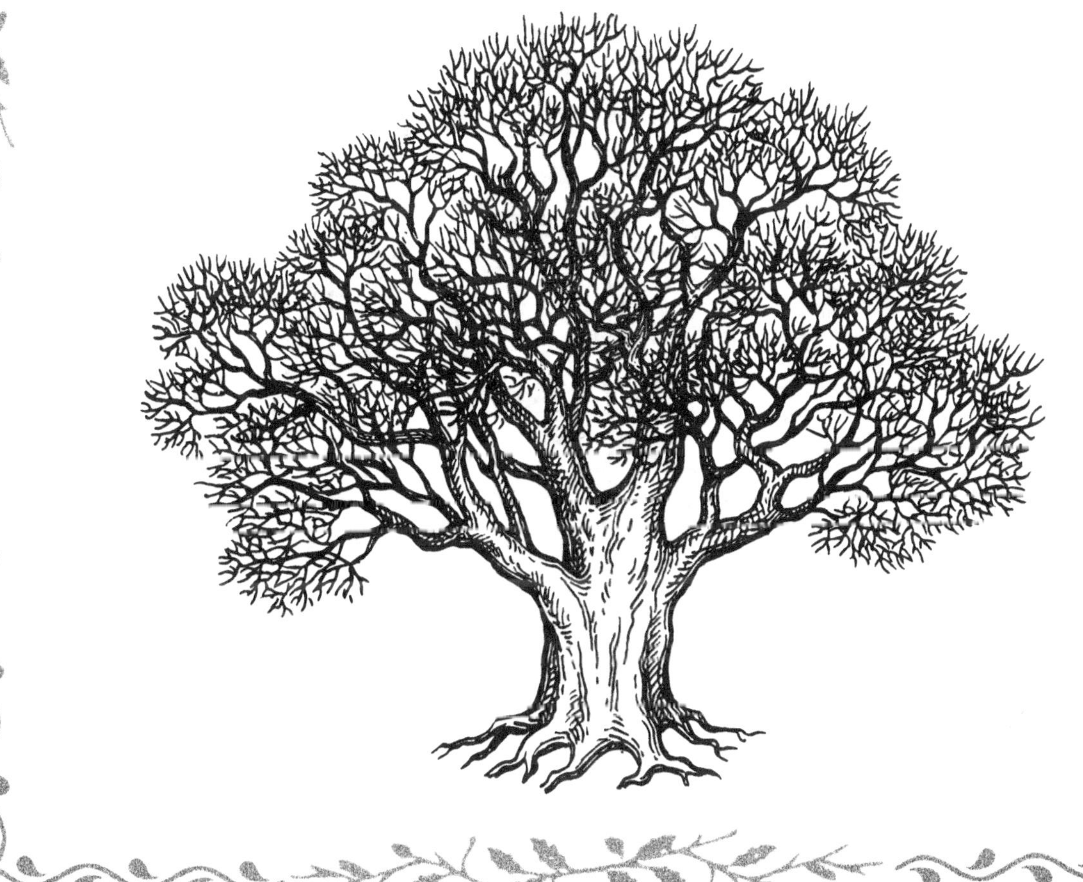

Cognitive Enrichment Activities:

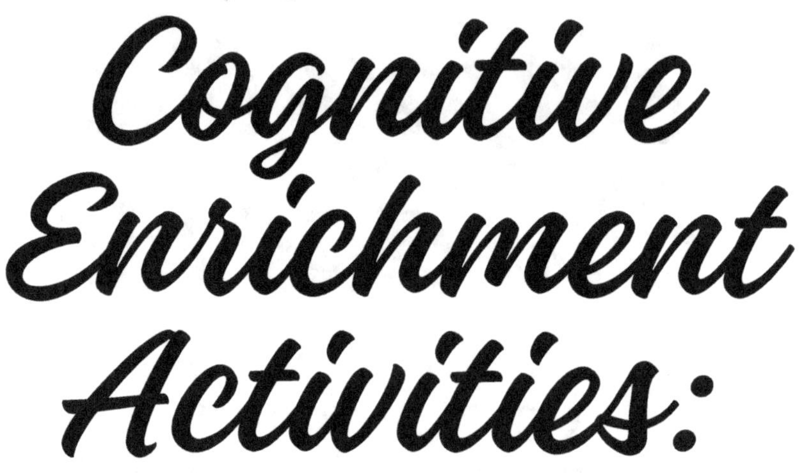

- Engage in activities that provide cognitive enrichment, such as attending lectures or joining book clubs.
- Intellectual stimulation contributes to cognitive vitality.

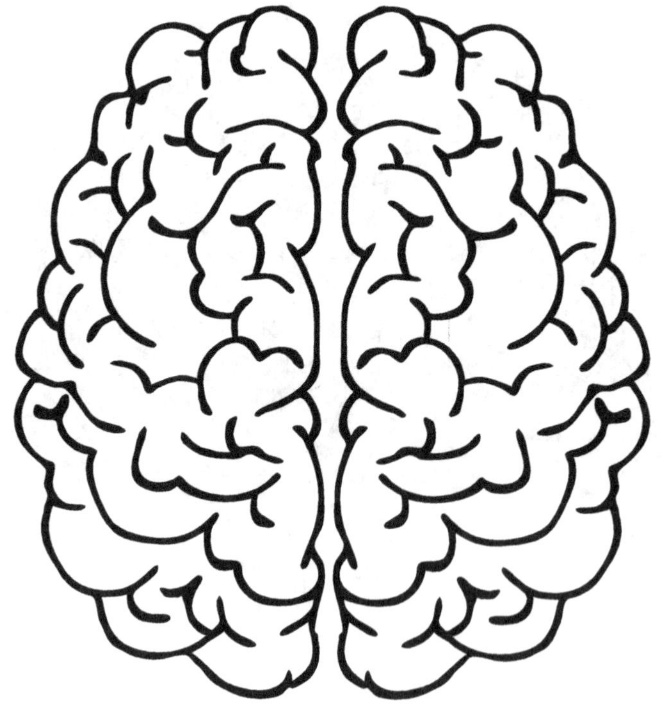

Stay Attuned to Emotions:

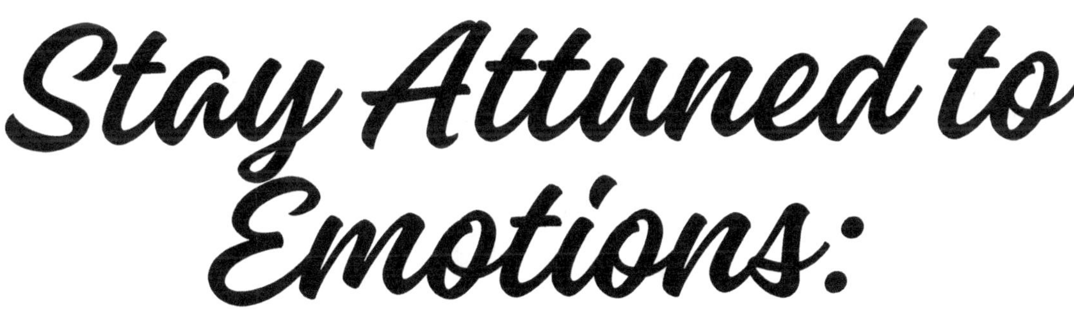

- Pay attention to your emotional well-being and seek support when facing emotional challenges.
- Emotional health is integral to overall well-being.

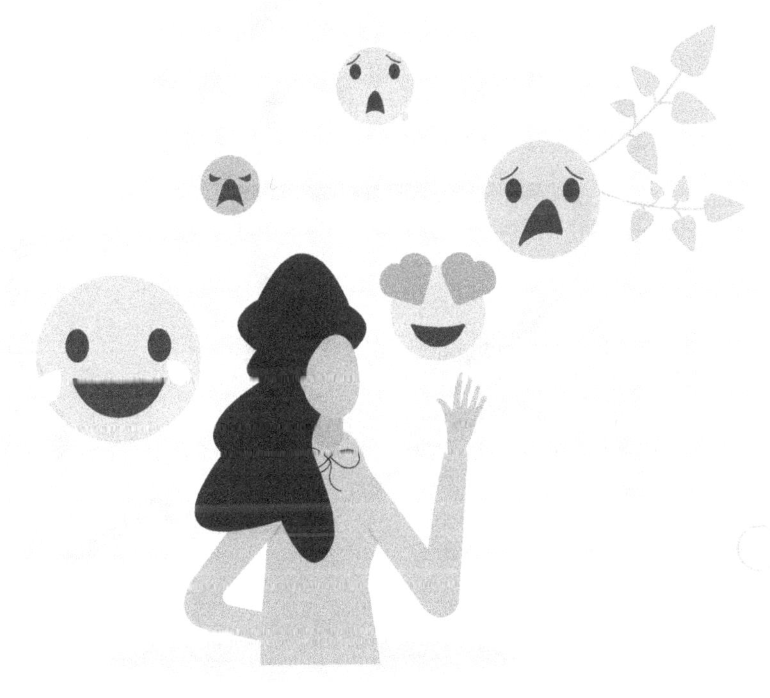

Laugh and Have Fun:

- Incorporate laughter and humor into your life.
- Whether through socializing, watching comedies, or engaging in activities that bring joy, laughter contributes to a positive outlook.

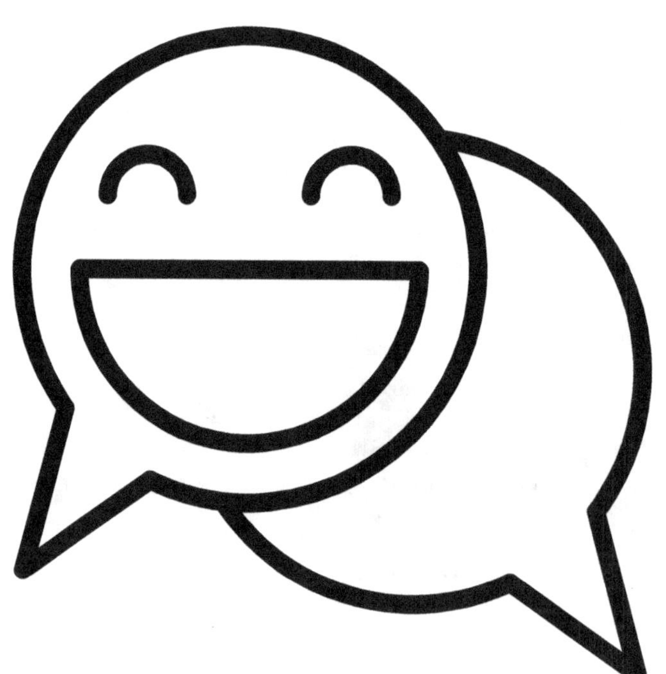

Explore Holistic Therapies:

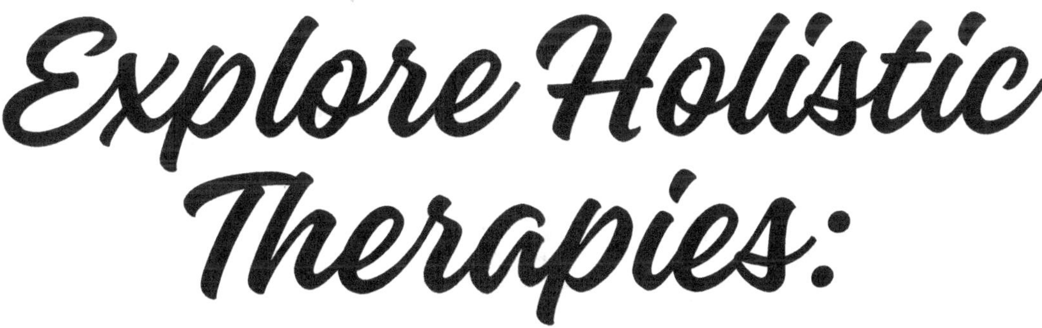

- Investigate holistic therapies such as aromatherapy, acupuncture, or herbal remedies.
- Consult with healthcare professionals to ensure these approaches align with your health goals.

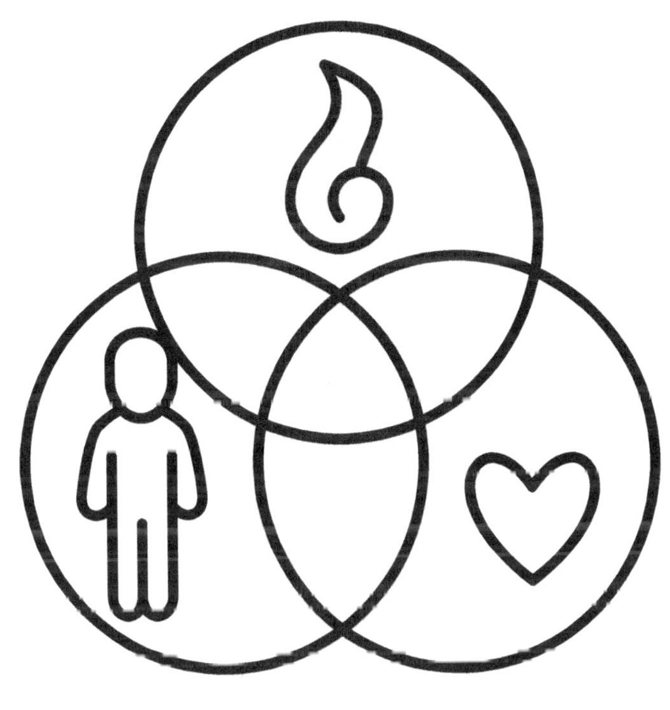

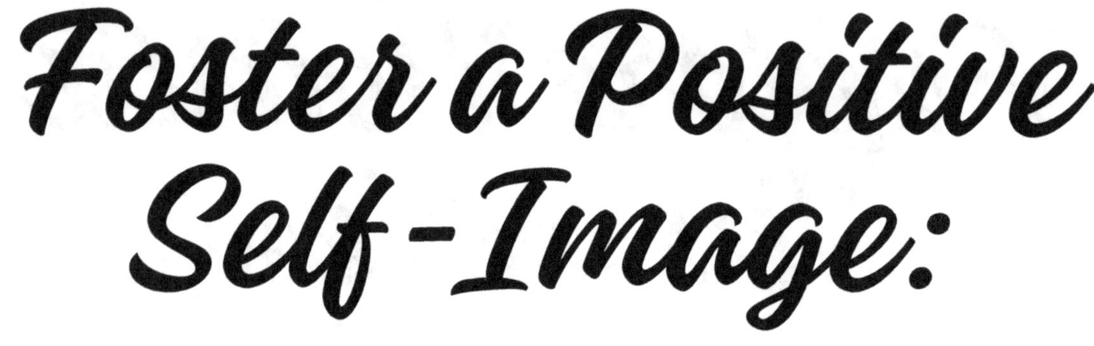

- Cultivate a positive self-image by focusing on your strengths and achievements.
- Surround yourself with positive influences that uplift and support you.

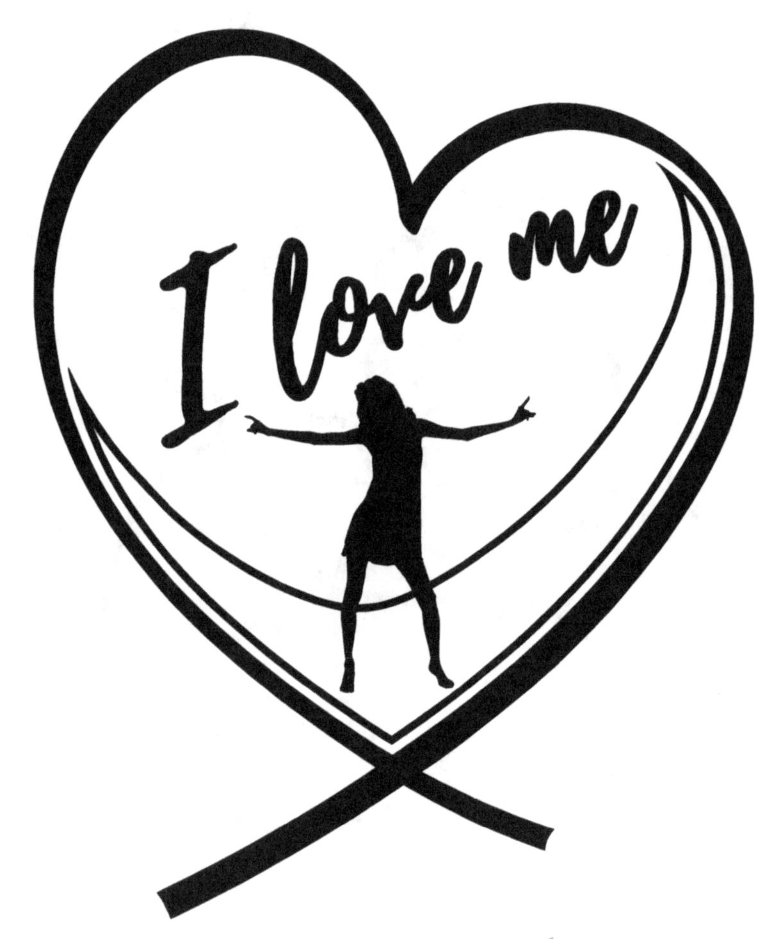

Travel Safely:

- If you enjoy travel, plan trips that cater to your comfort and safety.
- Consider accommodations that offer accessibility features, and check with your healthcare provider for travel recommendations.

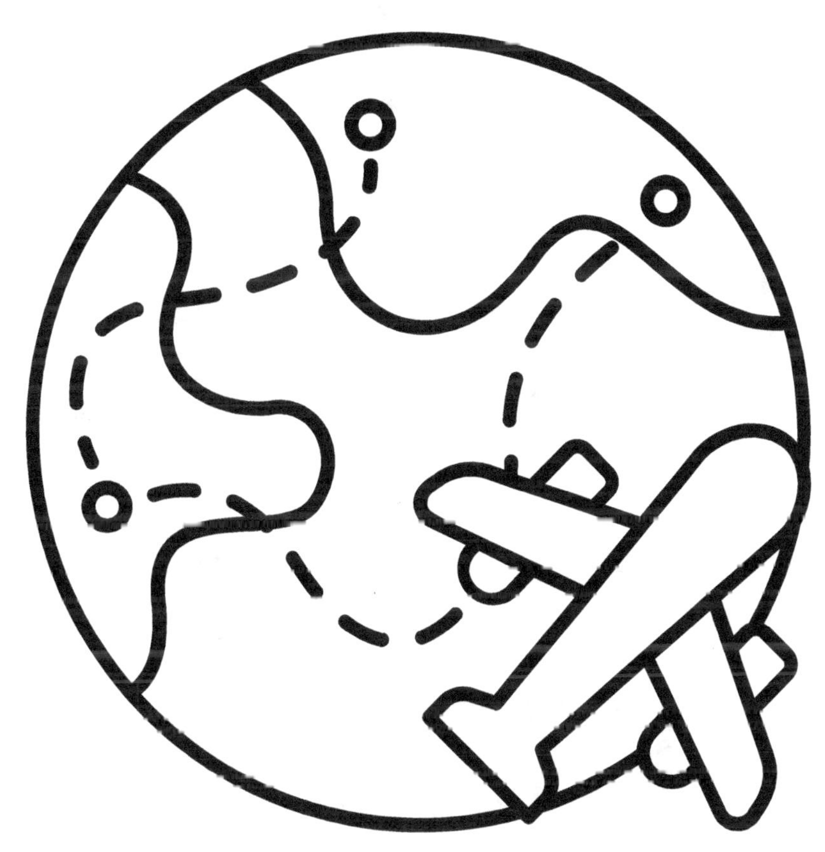

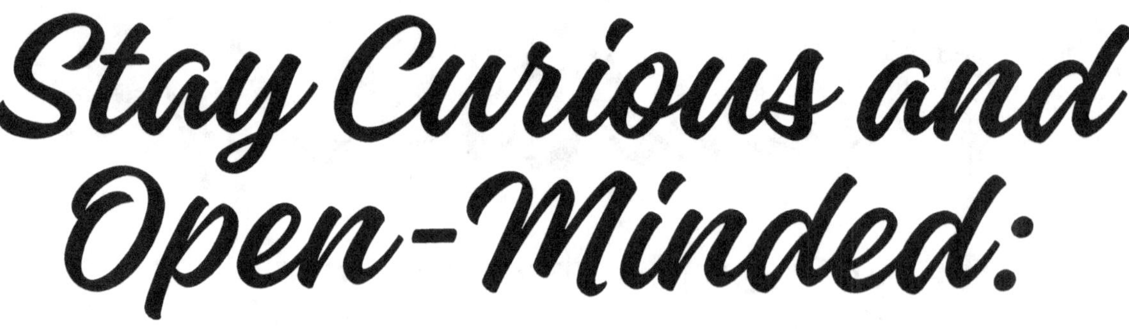

Stay Curious and Open-Minded:

- Cultivate a curious and open-minded attitude toward life.
- Embrace new experiences, ideas, and perspectives to keep your mind engaged and adaptive.

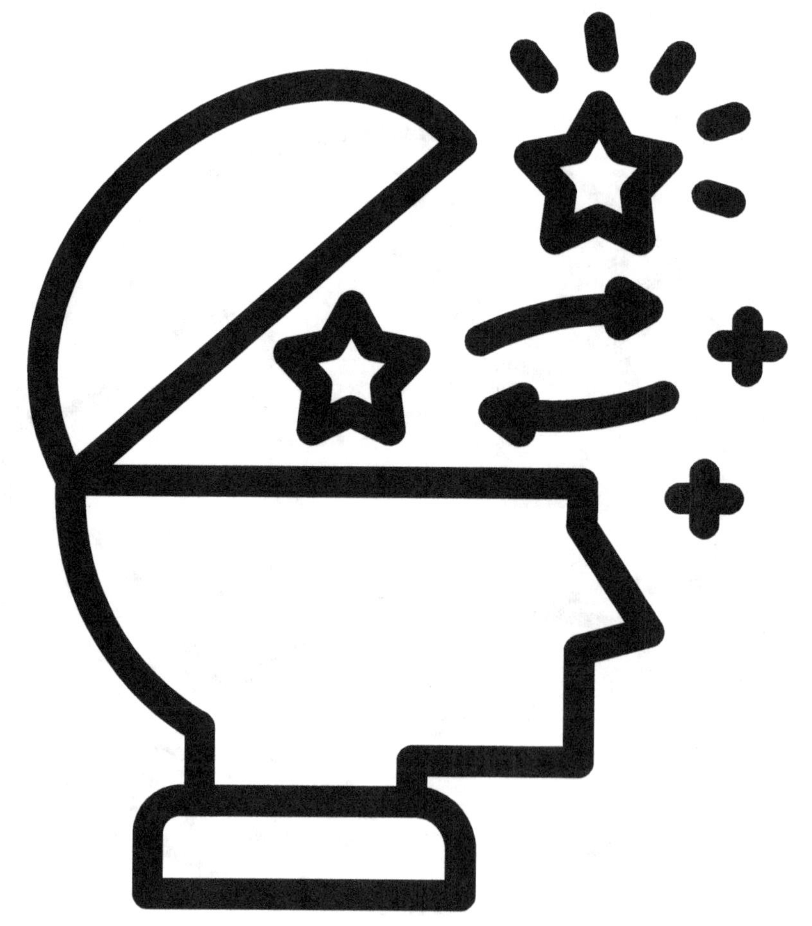

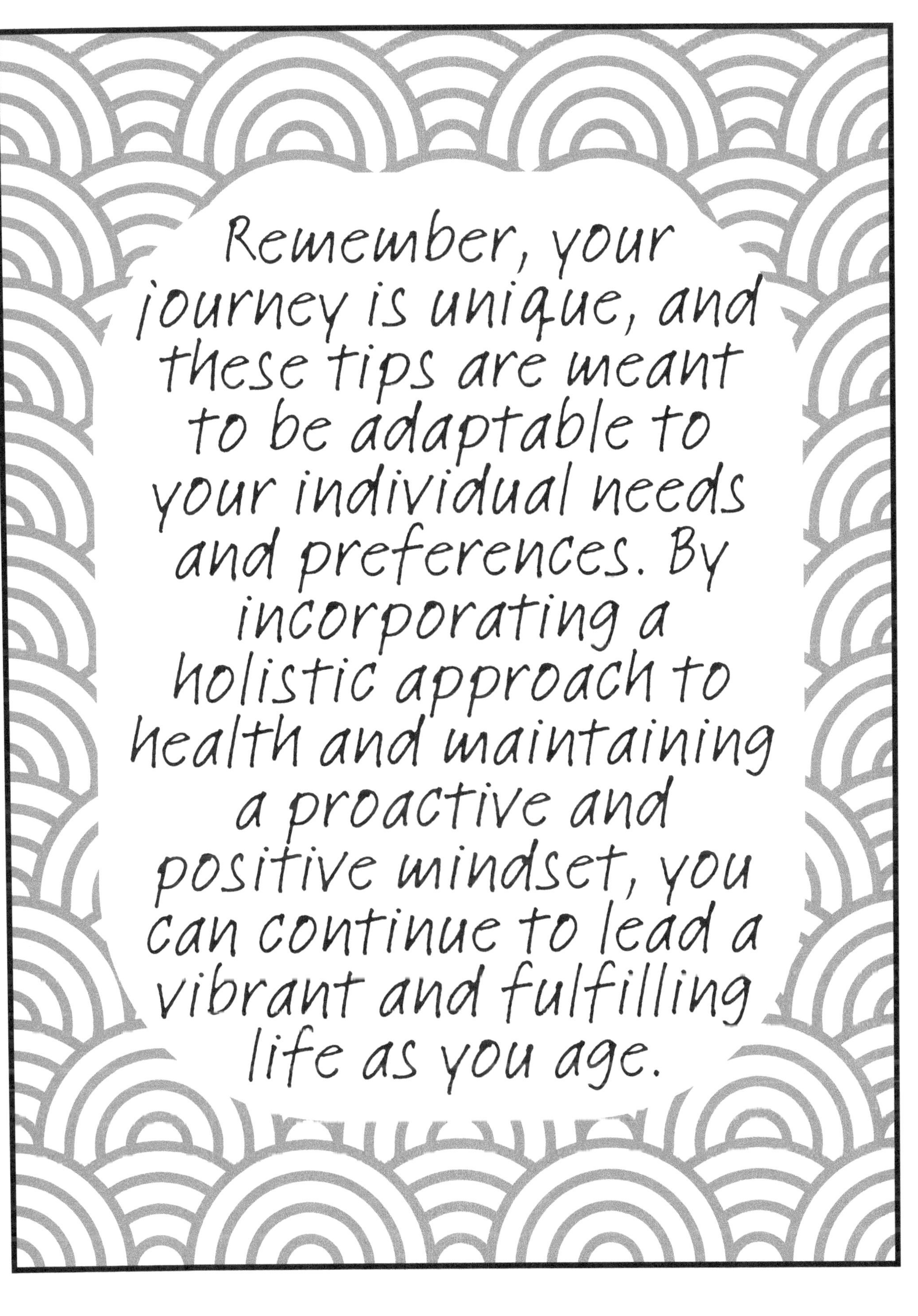

Remember, your journey is unique, and these tips are meant to be adaptable to your individual needs and preferences. By incorporating a holistic approach to health and maintaining a proactive and positive mindset, you can continue to lead a vibrant and fulfilling life as you age.